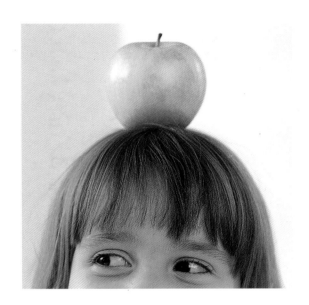

IMMUNITY FOODS FOR
HEALTHY KIDS

D1500495

To Max, Otto and India

IMMUNITY FOODS FOR HEALTHY KIDS
Lucy Burney

First published in 2004 by
Duncan Baird Publishers Ltd
Sixth Floor
Castle House
75–76 Wells Street
London W1T 3QH

Conceived, created and designed by Duncan Baird Publishers

Managing Editor: Rebecca Miles
Editorial Assistant: Emily Mason
Managing Designer: Manisha Patel
Designer: Adelle Morris
Commissioned Photography: William Lingwood
Children's Photography: Vanessa Davies
Stylists: David Morgan (food), Helen Trent

British Library Cataloguing-in-Publication Data:
A CIP record for this book is available from the British Library

ISBN-10: 1-84483-120-5   ISBN-13: 9-781844-831203

10 9 8 7 6 5 4 3 2 1

Typeset in Helvetica
Colour reproduction by Scanhouse, Malaysia
Printed and bound in Singapore by Imago

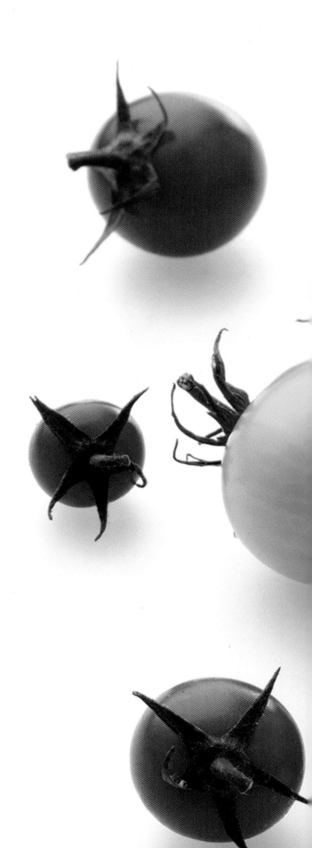

PUBLISHER'S NOTE: *Immunity Foods for Healthy Kids* is not intended as a replacement for
professional medical treatment and advice. The publishers and authors cannot accept
responsibility for any damage incurred as a result of any of the therapeutic methods
contained in this work. If you are suffering from a medical condition and are unsure of
the suitability of any of the therapeutic methods or food supplements mentioned in this
book, or if you are pregnant, it is advisable to consult a medical practitioner.
Essential oils must be diluted in a base oil before use. They should not be taken
internally and are for adult use only.

The abbreviation BCE is used in this book:
BCE Before the Common Era (the equivalent of BC)

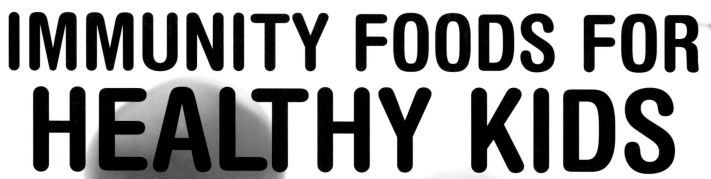

IMMUNITY FOODS FOR
HEALTHY KIDS

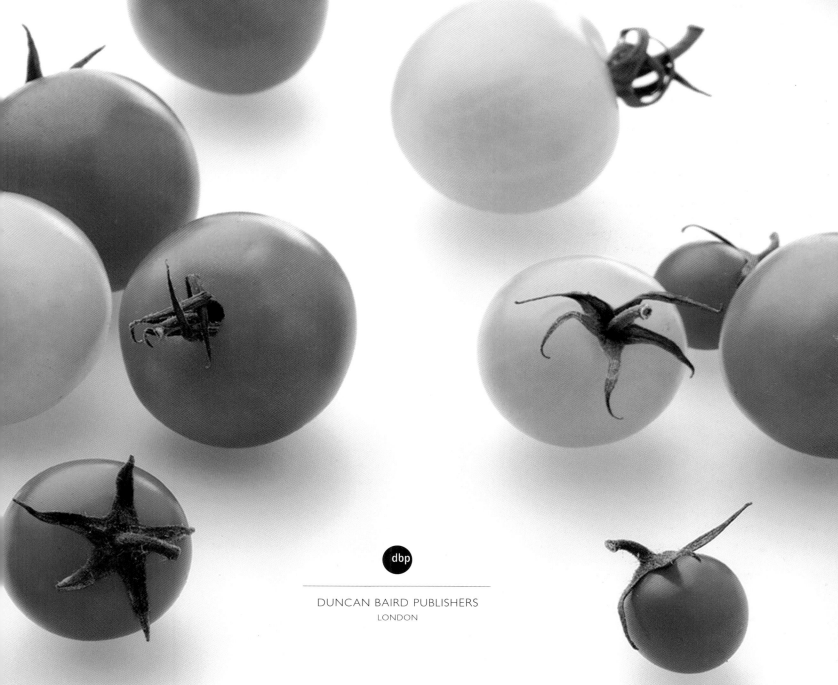

dbp

DUNCAN BAIRD PUBLISHERS
LONDON

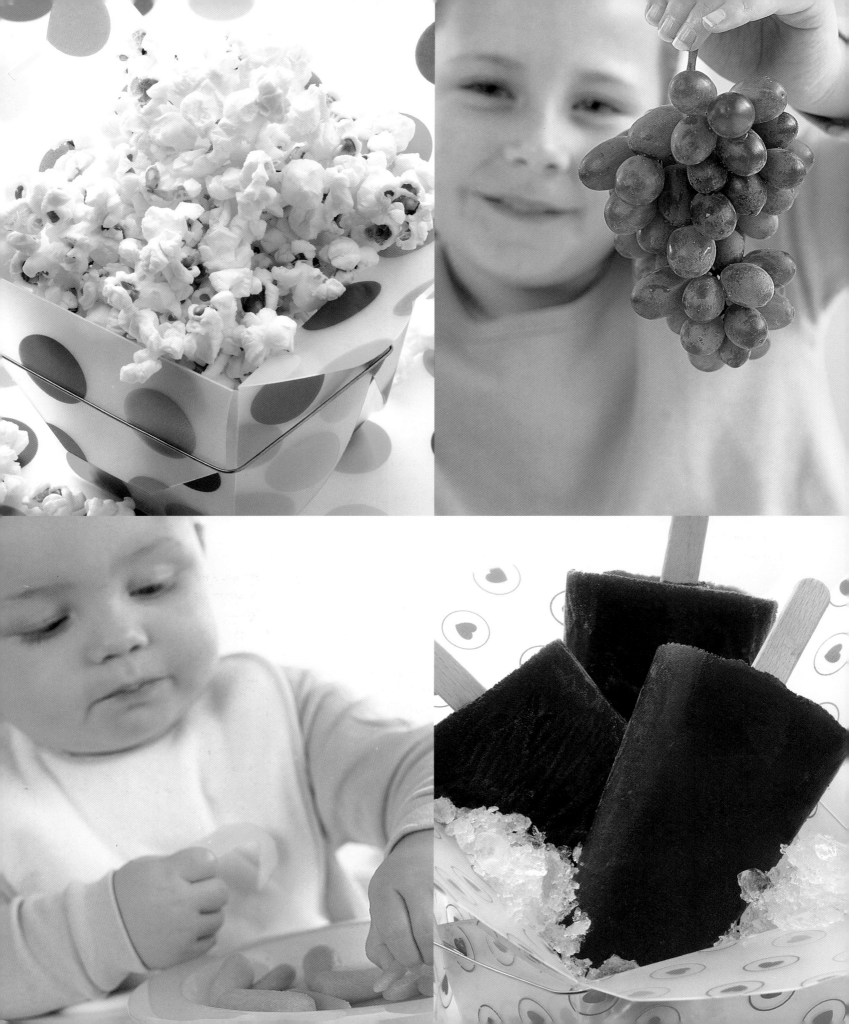

contents

Introduction 6

PART ONE:

Understanding Your Child's
Immune System 8

What is immunity? 10

How the immune system works 10

Building immunity the natural way 12

Allergy and autoimmunity 15

The vaccination dilemma 15

PART TWO:

Foods for Immunity 16

Salad vegetables 18

Root vegetables 19

    Star food: broccoli 20

Green leafy vegetables 22

    Star food: shiitake mushroom 24

Other vegetables 26

Summer fruits and berries 27

    Star food: blackcurrant 28

Everyday fruits 30

Exotic fruits 31

Dried fruits 33

    Star food: orange 34

Nuts and seeds 36

    Star food: walnut 38

Grains 40

    Star food: oats 42

Meat, fish and dairy 44

    Star food: game 46

    Star food: salmon 48

    Star food: yoghurt 50

Pulses and beans 52

Herbs, spices and condiments 53

    Star food: garlic 56

PART THREE:

Immunity Recipes for Children 58

0–6 months 60

(Breastfeeding recipes)

    Menu plans 61

    Breakfasts 62

    Main meals 62

    Puddings and baking 66

    Drink 66

6–12 months 68

    Menu plans 69

    First fruit and vegetable purées 70

    First cereals 72

    First protein purées 72

    Puddings 75

1–4 years 76

    Menu plans 77

    Breakfasts 78

    Main meals 79

    Puddings and baking 82

    Drinks 83

5–12 years 84

    Menu plans 85

    Breakfasts 86

    Main meals 86

    Puddings and baking 90

    Drinks 91

13–18 years 92

    Menu plans 93

    Breakfasts 94

    Main meals 94

    Puddings and baking 98

    Drinks 99

PART FOUR:

Foods to Fight Common
Illnesses 100

Asthma 102

Candida 104

Coughs 106

Chicken pox 108

Chronic fatigue syndrome 110

Eczema 112

Food allergies 114

Glandular fever 116

Hay fever 118

Headaches & migraines 120

Measles 122

Sore throats 124

Ear infections 126

Cancer 128

Diabetes 130

Coeliac disease 132

Other illnesses 134

Glossary 136

Essential Nutrients 138

Guide to Phytonutrients 139

Index 141

Bibliography 144

SYMBOLS USED IN THIS BOOK

★ IMPORTANT NUTRIENTS

▨ PHYTONUTRIENTS

✓ IMMUNE-BOOSTING ACTION
   AND OTHER BENEFICIAL
   PROPERTIES

! WARNING

▨ WHEAT-FREE

▨ GLUTEN-FREE

▨ DAIRY-FREE

▨ VEGETARIAN

▨ SUITABLE FOR BABIES OVER
   6 MONTHS

1+ SUITABLE FOR CHILDREN
   OVER 1 YEAR

2+ SUITABLE FOR CHILDREN
   OVER 2 YEARS

5+ SUITABLE FOR CHILDREN
   OVER 5 YEARS

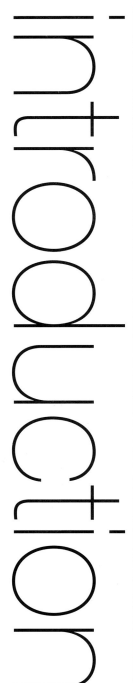

introduction

This book is all about your child's health and how and why it is affected by the food he eats. Health is not merely the absence of disease but a state of being that provides lifelong resistance to it. Your child's health is dependent on the development and maintenance of his immune system; and a strong, resilient immune system is created from the food and drink he consumes while growing and throughout life.

Nature possesses a treasure chest of nutrients that support and strengthen your child's defences. As well as the known essential nutrients required by the body, around 12,000 phytonutrients have recently been identified, with more being discovered each year. Phytonutrients, or phytochemicals as they are also known, are biologically active compounds that are found in plants and that promote health or prevent disease. Feeding your child a diet rich in phytonutrients will boost his immunity and enhance his general health.

Building a strong immune system for your child starts before he is even born, with the foods that his mother eats during pregnancy. These nourish the baby as the first few cells of his immune system are being formed in the womb. After birth, nature provides a true superfood for your child's immune system in breast milk. Rich in nutrients, it serves to feed and protect your baby from infection and allergies while his immune system starts to find its feet. As your baby grows and his immune system matures, you can introduce solid foods rich in antioxidants and phytochemicals that help to strengthen and nourish the immune army.

Your child's eating habits throughout his early years will set a dietary pattern for life. You will find that, during toddlerhood, he will come into contact with many viruses and bacteria. Nourishing him with an immune-boosting diet will help to protect him from infection and aid recovery in times of illness. During the school years and adolescence, your child will experience different pressures, and body changes, all of which can stress the immune system. Supplying a diet rich in nutrients that support the immune system is vital to help children and teenagers through this often difficult and unpredictable time. Also, as before, it will provide protection against childhood diseases and help overcome illness should it occur.

Optimum nutrition during times of illness is especially important. In this book you will find plenty of information and recipes to help speed your child's recovery from a variety of the most common childhood ailments and to harness his body's natural ability to heal itself.

As a mother as well as a nutritionist, I care passionately about children's health. My three children have had their fair share of colds, viruses and tummy bugs, but they have never had to take antibiotics and they exude a vitality that seems to be lacking in so many children. They are prepared to try any food that is put in front of them, as well as having their own personal likes and dislikes. I attribute this to the healthy and varied diet they have eaten all their young lives. As parents we are able to influence the strength of our children's immune systems through the food that we feed them. This book shows you how to give them the gift of health, both for now and for the future.

USING THIS BOOK

Immunity Foods for Healthy Kids offers a complete approach to your child's health through diet, focusing on the fundamental role played by the immune system. It is divided into four parts:

Part One, Understanding Your Child's Immune System, outlines the workings of your child's immune system. It gives clear, concise explanations of this complex subject, the details of which scientists believe we are only beginning to discover and understand.

Part Two, Foods for Immunity, looks in detail at 96 individual foods that can be beneficial to health when incorporated into your child's diet. Of these, ten "star foods" are highlighted as being particularly valuable to your child's immune strength.

Part Three, Immunity Recipes for Children, offers more than 100 recipes divided into five age groups: 0–6 months/breastfeeding, 6–12 months, 1–4 years, 5–12 years and 13–18 years. These will help you to feed your family nutrient-packed, immune-boosting meals from birth to adulthood.

Part Four, Foods to Fight Common Illnesses, describes some of the most common childhood ailments, how to recognize them and how to use certain foods to help alleviate symptoms and promote recovery.

profiles and symbols

Each of the foods described in Part Two is listed with an "immune profile" that is designed to give you an at-a-glance outline of the main nutritional benefits associated with it. The key to the symbols used in these profiles can be found on the contents page of this book. In addition, every main food entry is followed by a selection of some of the recipes found elsewhere in the book that feature the food as a principal ingredient.

Health-promoting recipes can be found throughout the book: alongside each "star food" in Part Two, divided into broad age-group selections in Part Three, and accompanying each childhood illness discussed in Part Four. To help those catering for children with common food allergies, under each recipe title you will see a line of symbols indicating whether or not the recipe is wheat-free, gluten-free, dairy-free or vegetarian and the age from which it is suitable to feed it to your child. The age-suitability for each recipe is based on the potential allergy risk of some of the ingredients and should be used in conjunction with your family's specific tastes and requirements – a recipe for stir-fried duck with orange and ginger may not contain anything harmful to a one-year-old but is pretty unlikely to appeal to their young tastes! The key to the recipe symbols can be found on the contents page of this book.

I recommend that you try to use organic produce whenever you can. This is especially important while weaning your baby, when I regard using organic food as imperative. Weight for weight, babies eat far more fruits and vegetables than adults and therefore their pesticide exposure from non-organic food is likely to exceed acceptable levels. Also, non-organic dairy products and meat contain potentially harmful residues of hormones and antibiotics routinely administered to animals, so are best avoided by an immature immune system as well.

I have used the pronouns "he" and "she" alternately in each part of this book. Hence, in Parts One and Three, "he" is used to describe children of both sexes, and in Parts Two and Four, I use "she".

Those who enjoy this book can find out more about children's health through my website www.lucyburney.co.uk There, you will be able to obtain new recipes, read the latest health news and discuss your concerns with other parents through my message board. You can email me directly in strictest confidence. I answer every email personally.

Lucy Burney

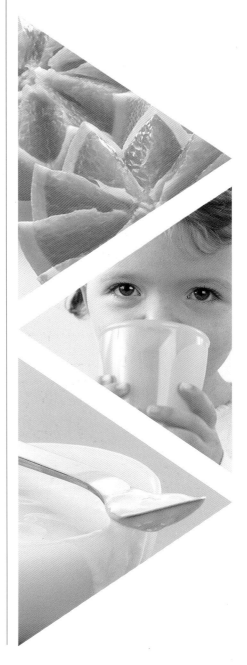

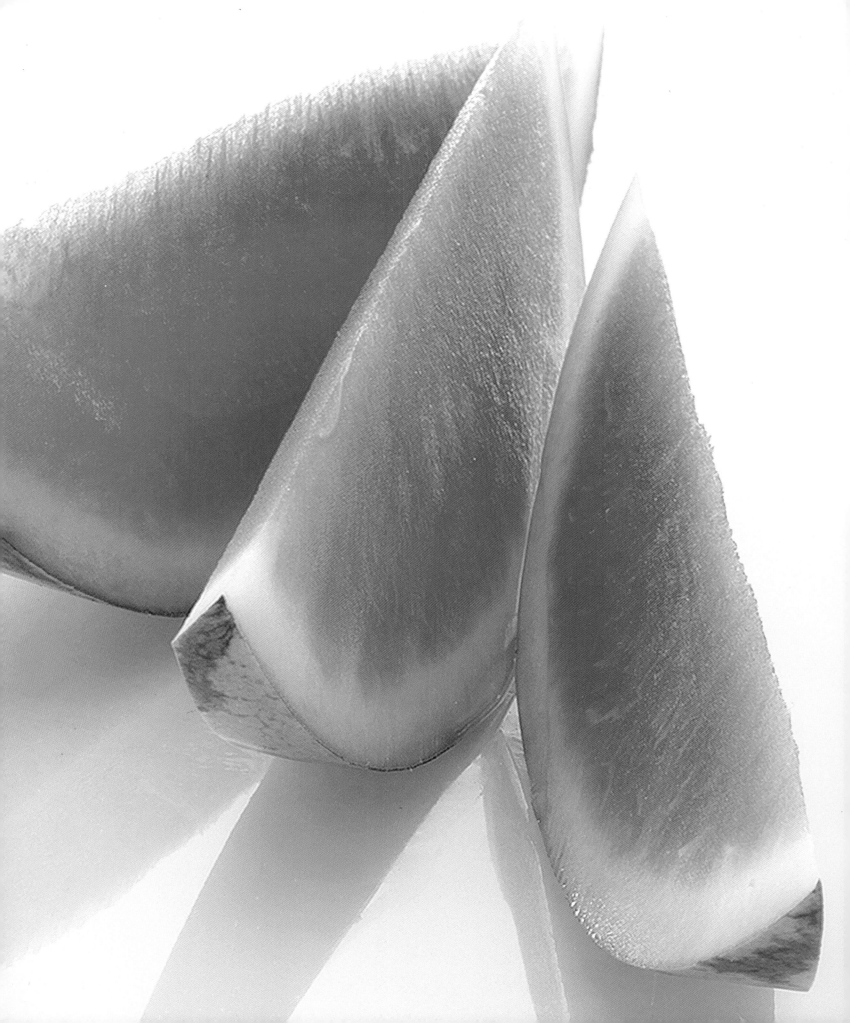

understanding your child's immune system

The key to a healthy child is a healthy immune system, and this, in turn, is developed and maintained by the food he eats. A sound knowledge of the workings of your child's immune system is vital if you are to support and nurture it throughout childhood. Part One contains all the information you need to fully understand your child's immune system – explaining how it matures throughout your child's life, how it protects against disease and how it sometimes goes wrong, either turning against itself, as in the cases of allergy or autoimmunity, or failing to protect the body from disease. We also examine the fundamental role of diet and nutrition in the maintenance of a strong immune system and address the controversial issues of vaccination and the use of antibiotics in the world today.

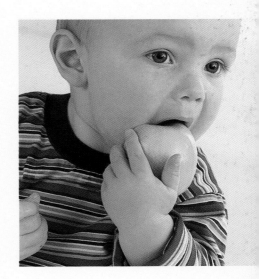

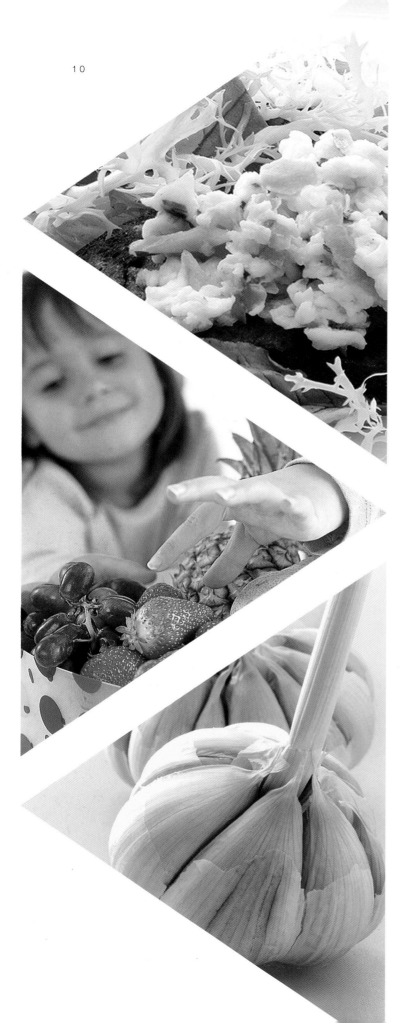

WHAT IS IMMUNITY?

Your child's immune system is his body's defence against infection, and immunity is the ability to resist infection. Every baby is born with a certain level of immunity, which has been passed on by the mother, via the placenta during pregnancy, and through breastfeeding thereafter. This is called passive immunity. However, from the ninth week of pregnancy onwards your baby's own immune cells are also forming, and his immune system is beginning to develop, although it is not considered fully mature until around the age of 14 years. This is why children are more susceptible to illnesses and infections during the initial years of their lives.

As well as being born with passive immunity, from birth onwards every child acquires active immunity through exposure to different infections. As part of this process, the immune system reacts against any invading germs by creating antibodies to kill them. Active immunity can be prompted by exposure to a virus, perhaps caught from another child at school, or by vaccination against a certain virus, such as measles. While the immune system is immature, it will gain strength after each and every encounter with germs. Every time it comes into contact with an infectious germ, the immune system stores the information so that it can remember and protect your child against it the next time it appears.

HOW THE IMMUNE SYSTEM WORKS

Your child's immune system is an incredibly complex, interactive system of organs, cells, chemicals and pathways that work together to form a defensive force against bacteria, viruses, fungi, parasites and other unwelcome germs. It works on three basic levels, or lines of defence. The first level is made up of some of the body's physical attributes. The skin is the body's most immediate defensive barrier, although it is by no means the largest in size. This award goes to the mucous membranes that line the respiratory, digestive and reproductive tracts, and have a surface area of around 400 square metres (4,300 square ft). Together, the skin and the mucous membranes form a massive external and internal barrier with the aim of preventing germs from gaining entry to the rest of the body. Other physical defence mechanisms include tears, sweat, urine, hydrochloric acid in the stomach, friendly bacteria in the gut and the tiny hairs that line the respiratory system. If any disease-causing organism does manage to breach this first line of defence, it has to contend with two further levels of the immune system, known as the innate immune system and the adaptive immune system.

the innate immune system

If bacteria manage to penetrate the immune system's first line of defence, through a cut, for example, the first division of the internal immune army, the innate immune system, automatically swings into action. One group of the body's white blood cells, macrophages, will rush to the site of any penetration to engulf and destroy the bacteria, often causing inflammation and swelling in the process. Other cells involved in this process are complement proteins, which can punch holes in bacteria cells thereby destroying them, and NK (natural killer) cells, a type of white blood cell that can destroy bacteria, parasites, virus-infected cells and cancer cells.

the adaptive immune system

If the innate immune system is overwhelmed or ineffective at repelling an invader, the third line of defence, the adaptive immune system, comes into play. Scientists believe that the human immune system has evolved this highly sophisticated system in order to protect our bodies against the more complex assaults mounted by viruses. White blood cells called lymphocytes that are produced by the bone marrow are the key cells at work here. To give some idea of their importance, an adult human has about a trillion lymphocytes present throughout the body, travelling around the lymphatic system (see below) and the bloodstream looking for invading germs.

Lymphocytes fall into two main categories: T-lymphocytes and B-lymphocytes. T-lymphocytes are further split into three types: T-helpers, T-suppressors and NK (natural killer) cells. The T-helpers stimulate the B-lymphocytes to produce antibodies and the T-suppressors tell the B-lymphocytes to stop this production once the invader has been identified and destroyed. The NK cells produce toxins capable of destroying identified invader cells and work with macrophages to kill them.

B-lymphocytes produce antibodies. Also known as immunoglobulins, antibodies are custom-made proteins secreted by the immune system in order to recognize and bind to a particular invader. They act as a tagging system, alerting other white cells to come and destroy the identified enemy. Once antibodies come into contact with a particular germ, they remember it, thus protecting the body against another attack later in life. If the germ returns, they recognize it and deploy a rapid response team to destroy it before it takes hold. There are five types of antibody:

● IgG is the main antibody, making up 75 per cent of the total produced by the immune system. It recognizes disease-causing microbes (pathogens) and is able to activate other proteins to destroy them. IgG is the antibody that passes most easily from the maternal placenta to the baby in the womb, supplying the unborn baby with protection that lasts into the first few months of life.

● IgA is the main antibody found in saliva, tears and the membranes of the digestive and respiratory tracts. IgA is also found in breast milk and helps to protect breastfed infants from gastrointestinal infection.

● IgE is the antibody involved in triggering allergic reactions. It stimulates the production of histamine, which is responsible for allergic symptoms, and is itself stimulated by allergens such as dust, pollen, insect bites or stings, pets, moulds and certain foods and drugs.

● IgM accounts for around 10 per cent of the body's antibodies. It is found in the bloodstream and is the first antibody to launch an attack when exposed to a potential pathogen. It is the main antibody created during infancy.

● IgD has recently been recognized as another type of antibody, albeit found in the body in very small amounts. Its specific role in the immune response has yet to be clarified.

the parts of the body making up the immune system

The central part of your child's immune system is the lymphatic system, a network of vein-like vessels running throughout the body that contains a clear liquid called lymph. In terms of transporting cells around the body, it is second in importance only to the cardiovascular system. Lymph is rich in T-lymphocytes and B-lymphocytes, the white blood cells that are key workers in the body's battle against infection. It is filtered through lymph nodes that are found in the neck, armpits, chest, abdomen and groin. These nodes produce and store lymphocytes as well as stimulating their activation. They also trap any unwanted invaders so that white blood cells can destroy them. Unlike blood, which is pumped around the circulatory system by the heart, lymph is propelled around the body by muscular movement because the lymphatic system does not have a pump. Instead, it relies on plenty of exercise to perform efficiently and can become sluggish with inactivity.

Elsewhere in the body, the thymus gland, bone marrow and spleen are also sites of white blood cell production and/or maturation. In addition, the tonsils, adenoids, appendix and parts of the small intestine known as Peyer's patches are important parts of lymphoid tissue and also provide protection against disease. Finally, although not technically part of the immune system, the liver plays an important supportive role by transforming many harmful substances, such as chemicals and pesticide residues, into harmless substances that can be excreted from the body as bile or urine.

BUILDING IMMUNITY THE NATURAL WAY

Given the right instruments, your child's body has a remarkable ability to heal itself. The immune army protects the body's boundaries and, once these have been penetrated, brings a plethora of strategies into play to protect your child from infection. In order to develop and thrive, your child's immune system needs to be nourished by the essential nutrients it requires to function efficiently. The chart below lists these key immune-boosting nutrients, their specific functions within the immune system, and tell-tale signs of deficiency.

All of these nutrients will be provided if your child is fed a diet filled with wholegrains, fruits, vegetables, lean meats, fish, nuts and seeds. Your child's immune system does not need a diet full of salt, sugar and saturated fat as this will seriously impede its function and lead to a higher risk of illness in later life.

IMMUNE-BOOSTING NUTRIENTS

nutrient	immune function	deficiency symptoms
VITAMIN A	Antioxidant; required for lymphocyte maturation and protection, maintenance of mucous membranes of respiratory, urinary and digestive systems, and essential fatty acid (EFA) metabolism	Dry skin, frequent infections, impaired growth, mouth ulcers, night blindness, poor hair condition
B-VITAMINS	Required for antibody formation, thymus development, lymphocyte production and EFA metabolism	Lack of energy, nervous disorders, poor hair, poor skin
VITAMIN C	Antibacterial; antihistamine; anti-inflammatory; antioxidant; antivrial; required for production of interferon, macrophage development and EFA metabolism	Allergies, bleeding gums, recurrent infections, slow wound healing
VITAMIN E	Antioxidant; required for antibody formation, protection of the thymus gland and EFA metabolism; works synergistically with selenium	Dry skin, easy bruising, slow wound healing
CALCIUM	Required for macrophage activity and fever production	Allergies, constipation, fatigue, hyperactivity, insomnia, irritability, muscle twitches
IRON	Required for production of white blood cells and antibodies	Anaemia, fatigue, intellectual impairment, intolerance of the cold, nausea, pale skin, poor appetite
MAGNESIUM	Required for antibody production, maintenance of thymus and EFA metabolism; controls histamine levels	Allergies, constipation, fatigue, hyperactivity, insomnia, irritability, muscle twitches
SELENIUM	Antioxidant; required for antibody formation and EFA metabolism; produces enzyme that kills cancer cells; works synergistically with vitamin E	Family history of cancer, frequent infections
ZINC	Antioxidant; required for lymphocyte development, EFA metabolism, and maintaining and protecting the thymus	Loss of taste and smell, poor appetite, poor growth, recurrent infections, white spots on nails

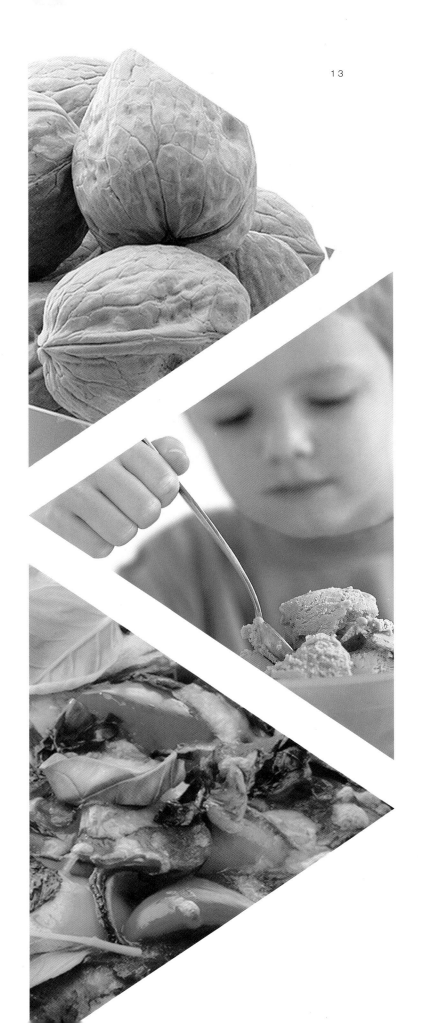

Further information on the general health benefits of the essential nutrients and their top food sources can be found in the chart on pages 138–9. In addition, each food entry in Part Two has an "immune profile" listing the essential nutrients that are present in significant quantities and any key phytonutrients that it has to offer. Phytonutrients are the substances derived from plant-based foods that have been found to excel in promoting certain aspects of health or in preventing certain diseases. See the chart on pages 139–40 for a list of the main phytonutrients mentioned in this book, their specific health benefits and rich food sources.

Some of the essential nutrients, and many of the phytonutrients, featured in this book have one common immune-boosting property – the fact that they are all antioxidants. This means that they help the body to fight any free radicals, which are molecules that can damage cells and cause disease. Free radicals are a by-product of combustion and occur as a result of the body's normal metabolism. They are usually kept in check by the antioxidants derived from a normal balanced diet. However, the production of free radicals can be increased by infection or by external environmental factors, such as pollution, radiation, burnt or fried food and cigarette smoke. Too many free radicals can cause disease, overwhelming and compromising your child's immune system. Eating foods especially rich in antioxidants combats any increase in their production, thus helping the body to fight illness. The key antioxidant nutrients are the vitamins A, C and E; the minerals zinc and selenium; and the carotenoid and flavonoid groups of phytonutrients. You can keep your child's immune system in optimum condition by regularly boosting their antioxidant intake. This is especially important in times of illness as antioxidants will significantly improve rates of recovery.

the role of antibiotics

As well as making sure that your child's diet equips him with a strong immune system to resist infection and boost general health, you also need to consider the role played today by antibiotics in fighting disease. It is clear that although antibiotics can be an effective agent in fighting bacterial disease, their prescription on such a huge scale over the past 50 years has caused some grave problems. Most illnesses to which children are exposed in their early years are viral, such as colds, coughs and chicken pox. If a bacterial infection occurs, it is usually secondary to the virus.

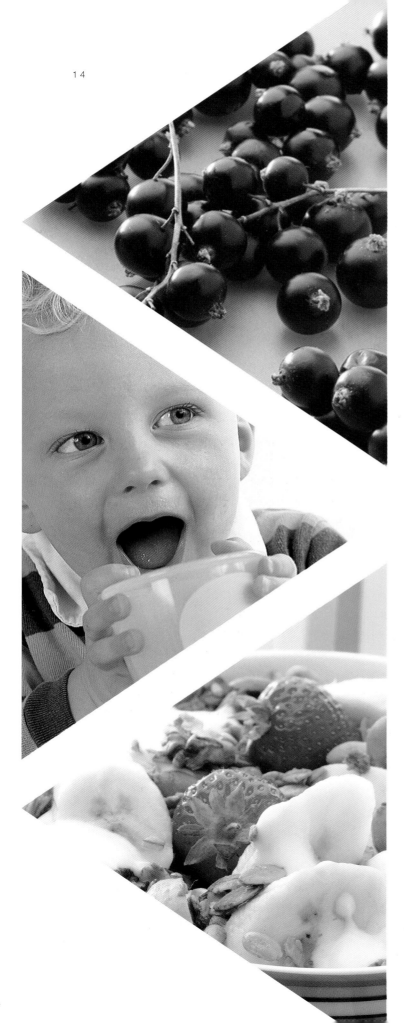

Antibiotics will work only against bacterial infections, not against viruses. They should never be prescribed for viral infections unless evidence of a bacterial infection is also present. Today, we are seeing a marked rise of antibiotic-resistant bacteria, caused by the widespread prescription, or over-prescription, of antibiotics in recent decades. These pose a serious threat, especially in hospitals, where an increasing number of patients die from a bacterial infection contracted in the hospital rather than from the illness or procedure for which they were first admitted.

Bacterial resistance is not only a result of the antibiotics that we take or give to our children. Our bodies are also absorbing residues of antibiotics from the non-organic meat and dairy products we consume. Bacteria adapt and mutate to develop stronger forms each time they come into contact with antibiotics, and the more frequent this exposure, the stronger they become. Diseases such as tuberculosis and diptheria, once thought of as controllable in the developed world, are on the increase, with some strains showing resistance to conventional antibiotic treatment. In addition, widespread routine use of antibiotics as part of intensive farming practices has led to a rise in antibiotic-resistant bacteria in animals, and evidence suggests that this is causing a cross-resistance from animal to human drugs. We need to reassess the way antibiotics are used and, as far as our children are concerned, use them only when absolutely necessary. In addition, we can make choices about the kinds of foods we feed our children – careful selection of a range of fresh, organic produce will doubtless boost their immune systems and help their bodies to combat any type of illness that might arise.

For viral infections, including colds and flu, your child needs bed rest, tender loving care and nourishment to support the body's fight against the infection. Every infection that your child contracts makes his immune system stronger. It needs this exposure to build up a memory of unwanted pathogens that are to be kept at bay. Illness in your children should not provoke the knee-jerk reaction of reaching for the medicine cupboard or calling the doctor. Clearly, however, there is a very important role to be played by the medical world, especially in the case of serious diseases such as meningitis where speed of treatment can make the difference between life and death. However, this is rare. Follow the recommendations covered in Part Four of this book to help nurture a sick child back to health and to support and strengthen his immune system along the way.

ALLERGY AND AUTOIMMUNITY

Unfortunately, the immune system does not always work according to plan. Things can, and do, go wrong. Sometimes it gets in a muddle and confuses the messages that it sends out to cells. The overall job of the immune system is to recognize what is "self" and what is not. It aims to destroy anything that is not "self" by launching an immune attack. Problems occur when your child's immune system identifies harmless substances or, worse still, useful substances, and launches an attack against them. When it attacks a harmless substance, such as flower pollen or a particular food, an allergic reaction can occur. When the immune system confuses "self" with "non-self" and launches an attack against useful cells in its own body, as in the case of rheumatoid arthritis or juvenile diabetes, this is called an autoimmune disease.

allergy

Allergies can develop at any age. Some occur in infancy while others can lay dormant for years without the person having any idea that they have an allergy at all. When your child first encounters an allergen that triggers an immune response, no symptoms occur. Instead the immune system becomes sensitized and creates a vast number of antibodies to fight that particular allergen on a future occasion. On further exposure to the allergen, for example an insect sting or a particular food or medication, the immune system goes into overdrive and releases chemicals that cause the inflammatory allergic symptoms of sneezing, coughing, wheezing and, in rare cases, anaphylactic shock.

Conventional treatment for allergies is to identify the allergen and try to reduce exposure to it, combined with orthodox medical treatment usually involving inhalers and bronchodilators. See pages 114–15 for information on how specific foods can help to treat allergy symptoms.

autoimmunity

Autoimmune diseases are not very common in childhood, but they are becoming increasingly common in teenagers. Juvenile diabetes (Type I), Crohn's disease, rheumatoid arthritis and ulcerative colitis are now occurring at a higher rate among teenagers than ever before. One hypothesis is that this is because of the low intake of essential fatty acids and the relatively high intake of saturated fat in the Western diet. The populations with the lowest rate of autoimmune diseases are those that eat a diet high in essential fats. Another theory is that exposure to certain viruses, or even vaccinations, may trigger a faulty immune response and result in the body attacking itself. In those that develop an autoimmune disease there is often a family history of the same or a different immune disorder.

THE VACCINATION DILEMMA

In most countries in the developed world, your baby will be due to have his first batch of immunisations against meningitis, diptheria, tetanus, whooping cough and polio at around eight weeks old. By the time your child goes to school, he will have received between 24 and 30 different vaccinations against measles, mumps, rubella, diptheria, tetanus, whooping cough, polio and meningitis. The precise number of vaccinations differs from country to country.

The aim of vaccination is to create artificial immunity to a certain disease. When your child catches an infectious viral disease such as chicken pox, his immune system springs into action, forming antibodies to that disease, and a battle ensues. Once the disease has been overcome, the antibodies remain to protect your child should he encounter the disease again. Vaccination is based on the premise that you can artificially create this immunity by injecting ready-made antibodies or so-called harmless versions of the micro-organism to stimulate your child's body to launch an assault and thereby create the desired antibodies to the disease.

The main controversy over vaccination is that little research has yet been carried out on the cocktail effect of vaccinations. At two months, your baby's immune system is undeveloped, still protected through passive immunity. Some healthcare professionals now believe that these immunizations, given at such a young age, can trigger immune malfunctions in susceptible children and that these can cause disastrous effects.

This is a highly emotive subject. Making choices regarding vaccination is a dilemma that every parent faces. There is no doubt that if you decide not to vaccinate your child, you take on a huge responsibility. To help you to decide, there is now plenty of literature available on the subject, covering every viewpoint. Whether or not you vaccinate, strengthening your child's immune system is something that every parent should know how to do. Following the guidelines set out in this book will help you to do so effectively.

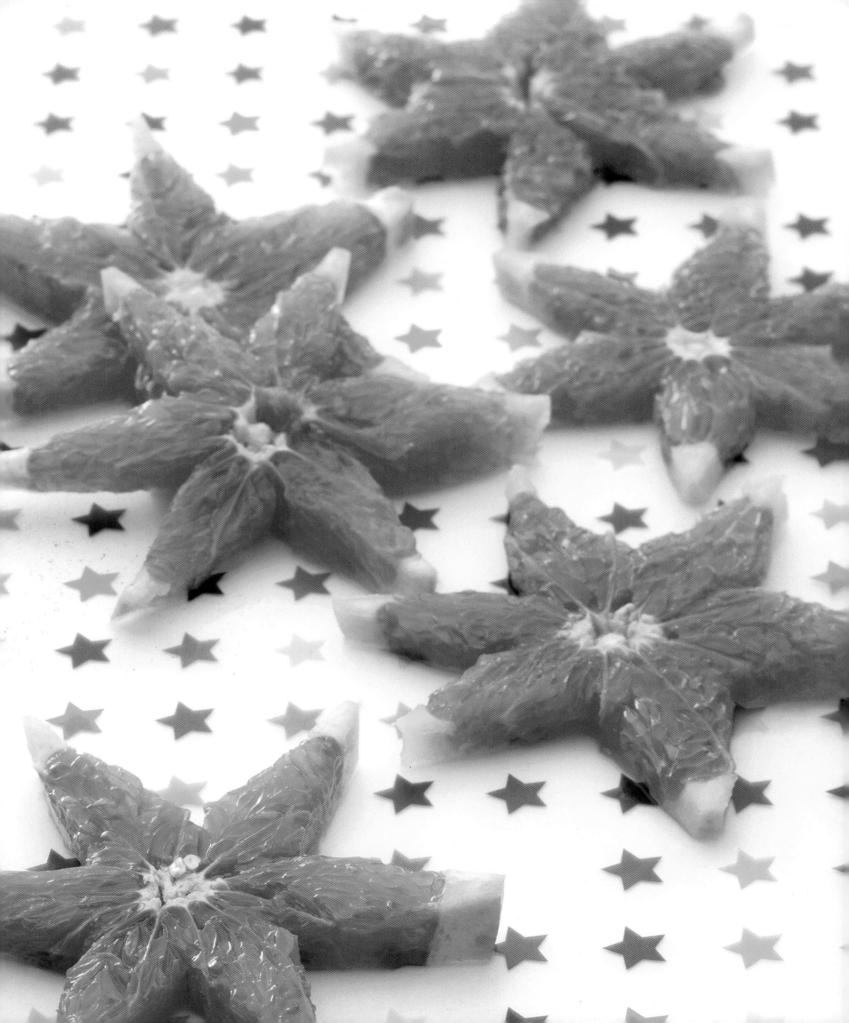

foods
for immunity

Many of the foods we eat have specific health benefits related to preventing illness and bolstering immunity. Part Two presents profiles of 96 foods, chosen because they are packed full of immune-boosting nutrients that help to protect your child from disease. The profiles also give information on the important phytonutrients in each food that give an extra boost to immune defences and can help to ward off everyday viruses. Included are ten "star foods", such as garlic and broccoli, which are of particular importance owing to their protective effects. Learn how to incorporate these foods into your child's diet and try out the accompanying recipes. As ever, these are easy to prepare and appeal to a wide range of age groups. Remember to check the recipe codes for potential allergy information and age suitability. All recipes serve four unless otherwise stated.

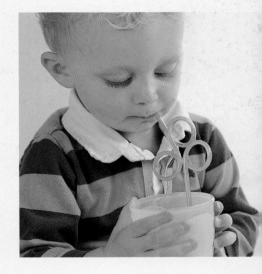

vegetables

SALAD VEGETABLES

AVOCADO

★ BETA-CAROTENE, VITAMINS C AND E; MAGNESIUM, POTASSIUM;
MONOUNSATURATED FAT

▨ ALPHA-CAROTENE

✓ ANTICARCINOGENIC, ANTIOXIDANT

Avocados are rich in the antioxidants beta-carotene and vitamins C
and E, which, like all antioxidants, combat free radicals and help to
protect your child's body from them. Free radicals are a chemical
by-product of the body's normal metabolic processes and can harm
cells, causing disease, if not kept in check. Free-radical production
can be boosted in times of infection, so antioxidant-rich foods are a
great help in overcoming illness. Avocado is easily digested and can
be an excellent weaning food. Combined with banana, it makes a
delicious purée full of essential nutrients for a growing baby.

*RECIPES: pine nut, avocado, red onion and watercress salad sandwich
(page 65); avocado and banana purée (page 70); fresh tomato, avocado and
pine nut pasta sauce with balsamic vinegar (page 97); guacamole (page 119)*

BEETROOT

★ BETA-CAROTENE, FOLIC ACID, VITAMIN C; CALCIUM, IRON, POTASSIUM

▨ CAROTENOIDS, FLAVONOIDS

✓ ANTICARCINOGENIC, ANTIOXIDANT

Beetroots are often a popular vegetable for babies and young
children as they have a high natural sugar content, which makes
them taste sweet. Rich in flavonoids and other anticarcinogenic
compounds, beetroots are an excellent immune-booster to include
in your child's diet. They are also a good source of folic acid and
potassium, both of which help maintain nervous-system health. As
well as the roots, beetroot tops can be eaten either cooked or
added to salads. These are rich in calcium, important for healthy
bones and teeth, and iron, which maintains energy levels and aids
the transportation of oxygen around the body in the blood. Don't
be alarmed if beetroot turns your child's urine pink. This is owing to
a natural red pigment called betacyanin, which is entirely harmless.

RECIPES: make your own pizza (page 80)

LETTUCE

★ BETA-CAROTENE, FOLIC ACID, VITAMIN C

▨ CHLOROPHYLL

✓ ANTICARCINOGENIC, ANTIOXIDANT

There are now so many varieties of lettuce on the market that you
can introduce your child to a wide selection from an early age. The
darker-coloured varieties contain the most nutrients, but even an
iceberg lettuce is a good source of folic acid, an essential vitamin
for a healthy nervous system. Beetroot tops, lollo rosso, Lamb's
lettuce, rocket, baby leaf spinach and romaine are just a few types
of lettuce that are rich in the disease-fighting antioxidants vitamin C
and beta-carotene. Once your child loves lettuce she will love it for
life. Find a dressing that she likes, full of essential fatty acids, to
complete an immune-boosting meal.

*RECIPES: family salads (page 81); hot salad with balsamic dressing and
fresh anchovies (page 98)*

PEPPERS

★ BETA-CAROTENE, VITAMIN C

▨ FLAVONOIDS

✓ ANTICARCINOGENIC, ANTIOXIDANT

Weight for weight, red and green peppers contain more vitamin C
than oranges and, along with beta-carotene, this powerful
antioxidant helps your child's body neutralize disease-causing free
radicals and can provide protection against cancer. Peppers are
also packed with flavonoids – immune-boosting phytonutrients with
antioxidant and antibacterial properties that amplify the food's
already strong antioxidant powers. Children tend to prefer red, yellow
and orange varieties of pepper to green, owing to their sweetness.

*RECIPES: roasted vegetables with coriander couscous (page 65); seafood
paella (page 66); family salads (page 81); gazpacho (page 94); queen
scallop stir-fry (page 98); family paella (page 98)*

TOMATO

★ BETA-CAROTENE, VITAMINS C AND E

▨ LYCOPENE

✓ ANTICARCINOGENIC, ANTIOXIDANT

Tomatoes are packed full of antioxidant vitamins, which help to protect your child's immune defences by boosting the fight against harmful free radicals. The vitamin C present in tomatoes also promotes skin health and wound healing and the vitamin E is good for blood-cell maintenance. Tomatoes are a rich source of the phytonutrient lycopene, which research suggests can prevent certain forms of cancer. Lycopene is present in both raw and cooked tomatoes. Tomatoes belong to the deadly nightshade family, which can cause allergic reactions in susceptible people. It is therefore wise to avoid tomatoes until the age of nine months.

RECIPES: roasted vegetables with coriander couscous (page 65); tempting tofu pasta sauce (page 74); my first pasta sauce (page 73); tuna and prawn brochette with coriander marinade (page 89); fresh tomato, avocado and pine nut pasta sauce with balsamic vinegar (page 97); mixed bean stew (page 131)

WATERCRESS

★ **BETA-CAROTENE, VITAMINS C AND E; CALCIUM, IRON**

▨ **CHLOROPHYLL, ISOTHIOCYANATES**

✓ **ANTICARCINOGENIC, ANTIOXIDANT**

Watercress is a great source of antioxidant vitamins, which help to strengthen your child's immune system. Particularly, it helps protect against colds and throat infections. It also contains iron, which stimulates the immune system, helps carry oxygen around the body and prevents anaemia. Watercress can have a hot, peppery taste so is better served to children in small amounts, perhaps as part of a salad or blended into a soup.

RECIPES: watercress soup (page 63); pine nut, avocado, red onion and watercress salad sandwich (page 65)

ROOT VEGETABLES

CARROT

★ **BETA-CAROTENE; FIBRE**

▨ **CAROTENOIDS**

✓ **ANTICARCINOGENIC, ANTIOXIDANT**

Children through the years have grown up being told that carrots help them to see in the dark. This is indeed true, owing to the exceptionally high levels

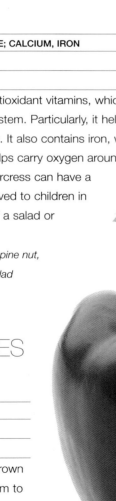

of beta-carotene contained in this vegetable. Your child's body converts beta-carotene (which is found only in plant foods) into vitamin A. As well as having potent antioxidant qualities, vitamin A is needed for healthy skin and vision and a deficiency symptom is night blindness. Carrots are also rich in fibre, which is important for the health of your child's bowel and digestive system. The therapeutic attributes of carrots have been well documented through the centuries. Puréed carrot has been shown to relieve diarrhoea in babies, whereas raw carrots can ease constipation both in children and adults.

RECIPES: my first carrot purée (page 70); my first pasta sauce (page 73); venison shepherd's pie (page 74); carrot and cashew nut soup (page 80); chicken and almond satay with carrot and sesame stir-fry (page 88); apple and carrot tonic (page 123)

broccoli

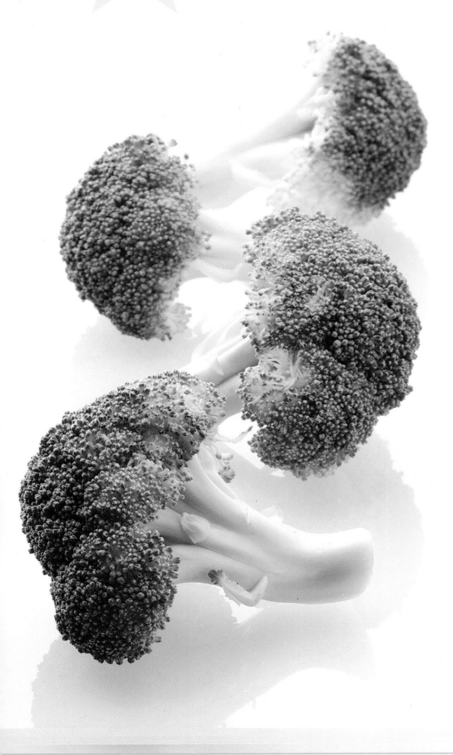

BROCCOLI IS A DELICIOUS AND VERSATILE VEGETABLE RICH IN ANTIOXIDANT VITAMINS AND PHYTONUTRIENTS THAT HELP TO PROTECT YOUR CHILD FROM DISEASE.

Origins

Broccoli *(Brassica oleracea)* is a dark green vegetable consisting of a dark green stalk that branches out at the end into florets. It can be green, purple or a deep blue-green. The name originates from the Latin *brachium*, which means arm or branch. Broccoli is a member of the cruciferous family of vegetables. Other members include cabbage, cauliflower, kale, bok choi, radish, turnip, watercress and Brussels sprouts. Cruciferous vegetables are well known for their substantial nutritional value. The first recorded mention of broccoli dates from Roman times when it was cultivated from wild cabbage that grew along the coasts of Europe. The vegetable reached England in the 1700s, probably coming from Italy as it was known as "Italian asparagus". Italian immigrants took broccoli to the United States around the beginning of the 1800s.

Immune-boosting profile

Broccoli is packed with immune-boosting nutrients and should feature regularly in your child's diet. Weight for weight, broccoli contains more vitamin C than oranges. Vitamin C is a powerful antioxidant that helps to protect against colds and other viral infections. It is also a free radical scavenger recognized for its ability to prevent the development of certain forms of cancer, as well as inhibiting the progress of HIV (Human Immunodeficiency Virus). In addition, vitamin C is required for the production of collagen, an important component of connective tissue. Your child's body is unable to create vitamin C for itself and has to obtain it through food.

Broccoli also contains the antioxidant beta-carotene, which has been identified as playing an important role in disease prevention. Beta-carotene belongs to the group of phytonutrients known as carotenoids (see page 139). Of 600 identified carotenoids, six (including beta-carotene) are particularly beneficial to health and incorporating them into the diet can reduce the risk of common diseases, such as heart disease, cancer and Type 2 diabetes. These six carotenoids also work synergistically with other antioxidants, such as vitamin C, to provide a better level of protection.

Broccoli is a good source of iron, too, which supports the production of white blood cells and antibodies, part of your child's immune army (see page 11). Without enough iron your child is more likely to suffer from frequent colds and other viral infections. Iron is a mineral that is often lacking in the toddler and pubescent diet causing the deficiency disease anaemia. Symptoms of anaemia are fatigue, pale skin, loss of appetite, nausea and sensitivity to cold.

Along with the other members of the cruciferous family, broccoli contains important sulphur compounds believed to protect against cancer, particularly of the bowel, stomach, breasts, kidneys and lungs. Broccoli is an excellent source of sulphoraphane, a phytonutrient with the ability to inhibit the production of cancer cells by activating one of the body's detoxification systems. The sprouts found on purple sprouting broccoli are a particularly good source – recent research has revealed that they contain as much as 20 times more sulphoraphane than green broccoli florets.

Using broccoli in your child's diet

Broccoli is one of the few green vegetables that seems to have universal appeal to children and is a great one to introduce to your child early on. It can be combined with other vegetables to make enticing purées for a baby. Toddlers are often happy to pick up broccoli "trees" as part of a meal and older children might enjoy florets eaten raw, or lightly steamed with dips. Also, broccoli sprouts make a great addition to a salad or sandwich.

The way you cook broccoli has a profound effect on its health-promoting qualities. Steaming or serving broccoli raw is far preferable to boiling, as boiled broccoli can lose more than half of its water-soluble vitamins along with its vibrant colour. Broccoli florets make a colourful addition to a stir-fry and, lightly steamed, they can accompany any main dish.

IMMUNE PROFILE

★ BETA-CAROTENE, FOLIC ACID, VITAMIN C; CALCIUM, IRON, POTASSIUM

▨ CHLOROPHYLL, FLAVONOIDS, INDOLES, SULPHORAPHANE

✓ ANTICARCINOGENIC, ANTIOXIDANT

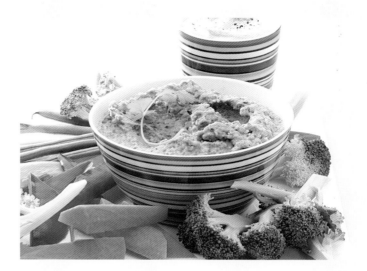

broccoli trees with crudités & dips *(above)*

This makes an excellent healthy snack for hungry schoolchildren. Lay out a large plate of crudités with some interesting dips for them to dive into when they get home.

1 small head of dark green broccoli, cut into small florets
1 carrot, peeled and chopped into matchsticks
A handful of raw French beans, washed and topped and tailed
½ cucumber cut into strips
1 red and 1 yellow pepper, deseeded and cut into big strips
2 sticks celery, cut into matchsticks

BEANY DIP
1 tin of mixed pulses, drained and rinsed in filtered water
1 garlic clove
A handful of fresh coriander
¼ cup extra virgin olive oil

In a food processor, blend all the ingredients together apart from the olive oil. Slowly drizzle the olive oil through the feeder at the top of the processor until you reach the desired consistency.

QUICK AND EASY HUMMUS
1 tin of chickpeas (no-sugar, no-salt variety)
2 garlic cloves
1 tbsp light tahini
8 tbsp extra virgin olive oil
1 tsp cumin seeds, ground
2 tbsp soya yoghurt (or live natural yoghurt if dairy-tolerant)
Black pepper to taste

Whizz all the ingredients together in a food processor.

CRUNCHY NUT DIP
2 tbsp almond butter
1 tbsp soya yoghurt (or live natural yoghurt if dairy-tolerant)
A squeeze of lemon juice

Mix the ingredients together and serve in a ramekin dish. Try also Anchoiade and Aioli (page 57) and Smoked Mackerel Dip (page 96).

ONION FAMILY

★ VITAMINS B1 AND B6; SULPHUR COMPOUNDS

▨ ALLICIN, QUERCETIN

✓ ANTIBIOTIC, ANTICARCINOGENIC, ANTI-INFLAMMATORY, ANTIVIRAL

Onions, garlic, chives, leeks and shallots all belong to the allium family. This group of vegetables has been revered for its therapeutic qualities for centuries. Onions contain phytonutrients that act as natural antibiotics, and garlic (see pages 56–7) has both antibacterial and antiviral properties. Researchers have also found that the sulphur compounds naturally occuring in onions may prevent the growth of cancer cells. These compounds are most active when the vegetable is raw: add onions to salads, salad dressings and soups to gain their maximum nutritional benefit.

RECIPES: watercress soup (page 63); pine nut, avocado, red onion and watercress salad sandwich (page 65); immune-boosting lentil purée (page 73); tuna fishcakes (page 79); quick and easy beany bake (page 80); the very best vegetarian burgers (page 86); egg and veggie bake (page 90); gazpacho (page 94); shiitake, spring onion and bok choi stir-fry with quinoa (page 111); immunity soup (page 123)

PARSNIP

★ FOLIC ACID, VITAMINS C AND E; FIBRE

✓ ANTICARCINOGENIC, ANTIOXIDANT

Parsnips are a popular root vegetable with children and can be a tasty alternative to potato in some recipes. They are rich in the antioxidant vitamins C and E, which help the immune system to fight disease-causing free radicals, and in folic acid, which plays a vital role in the growth and development of a healthy nervous system. They also contain plenty of dietary fibre, which is good for bowel health. Parsnips can be grated raw and added to salads or coleslaws. They are also delicious puréed or as part of a vegetable stew, and parsnips roasted in olive oil, garlic and rosemary make a wonderful addition to a traditional roast dinner.

RECIPES: chicken casserole (page 72)

POTATO

★ VITAMINS B6 AND C; POTASSIUM; FIBRE

✓ ANTICARCINOGENIC, ANTIOXIDANT

Potatoes are a great food staple and come in dozens of varieties. They provide a low-fat source of energy and dietary fibre and are a useful source of the antioxidant vitamin C, which helps to protect your child against infection. Potatoes also contain potassium, which helps maintain healthy nerves and muscles, and vitamin B6, which aids the production of haemoglobin, the part of red blood cells that carries oxygen around the body. Potatoes are highly versatile and can be baked, boiled, mashed or made into homemade chips.

RECIPES: warming lentil and potato bake (page 64); venison shepherd's pie (page 74); toddler fish pie (page 79); quick and easy beany bake (page 80); farmhouse lentil pie (page 82); venison sausages with pea, mint and potato mash (page 88); vegetable frittata (page 96); potato pizza (page 105)

SWEET POTATO

★ BETA-CAROTENE, VITAMINS C AND E

▨ CAROTENOIDS

✓ ANTICARCINOGENIC, ANTIOXIDANT

Originally from Central America, sweet potatoes are packed with antioxidant vitamins and phytonutrients; the richer their colour the more antioxidants they contain. These antioxidants help your child's immune system to combat disease. Sweet potatoes (which are unrelated to potatoes) make an excellent weaning food for babies as they taste sweet and have a very low allergic potential. For older children, you can drizzle them with olive oil, sprinkle with rosemary and bake them to make delicious homemade chips.

RECIPES: vegetable medley (page 70); cod and veggies (page 73); sweet potato and tahini (page 74)

GREEN LEAFY VEGETABLES

BOK CHOI (PAK CHOI)

★ BETA-CAROTENE, FOLIC ACID, VITAMIN C; POTASSIUM

▨ CHLOROPHYLL, ISOTHIOCYANATES

✓ ANTICARCINOGENIC, ANTIOXIDANT

Bok choi is a variety of Chinese cabbage that belongs to the same family of vegetables as broccoli, Brussels sprouts and other cabbages. It is an excellent source of the immune-protective antioxidants beta-carotene and vitamin C, and contains a range of phytonutrients that are believed to be cancer protective. Bok choi has white stalks with dark green rounded leaves and is usually sliced before cooking. Baby bok choi (sometimes called pak choi) are cooked whole. Stir-frying is the best method of cooking this vegetable and one that helps to preserve its nutrient content.

RECIPES: sweet and sour prawn stir-fry with egg noodles and bok choi (page 96); shiitake, spring onion and bok choi stir-fry with quinoa (page 111)

CAULIFLOWER

★ FOLIC ACID, VITAMINS B3 AND C

▨ SOTHIOCYANATES

✓ ANTICARCINOGENIC, ANTIOXIDANT

Cauliflower is a good source of vitamin C, the all-round immune-boosting vitamin that helps your child ward off viruses and infection. Vitamin C also aids iron absorption and promotes general skin health and wound healing. Vitamin B3, another essential nutrient present in cauliflower, similarly supports the health of the skin as well as helping to balance blood sugar levels. Cauliflower also contains members of the isothiocyanate group of phytonutrients, and these are believed to be especially anticarcinogenic and immune-protective. To preserve its maximum nutrient content, avoid boiling cauliflower. Instead, offer it raw with dips, lightly steamed or stir-fried.

RECIPES: *coconut and cauliflower soup (page 63); vegetable combos (page 70)*

GREEN AND RED CABBAGE

★ BETA-CAROTENE, FOLIC ACID, VITAMINS B3, C, E AND K

▨ ISOTHIOCYANATES

✓ ANTICARCINOGENIC, ANTI-INFLAMMATORY, ANTIOXIDANT, ANTISEPTIC

Cabbage is a nutrient-rich vegetable packed with the antioxidants beta-carotene and vitamins C and E. These help to strengthen the immune system and make cabbage a good seasonal vegetable to incorporate in your child's diet in the winter, when many colds and infections are around. It is also a valuable source of vitamin K, vital for normal blood clotting, and vitamin B3, which keeps skin healthy. Cabbage contains phytonutrients considered to protect against cancer. In addition, red cabbage is believed to have natural antiseptic substances. It is best to serve cabbage shredded and raw in a coleslaw, steamed or lightly stir-fried to preserve its vitamin content.

RECIPES: *Vegetable combos (page 70)*

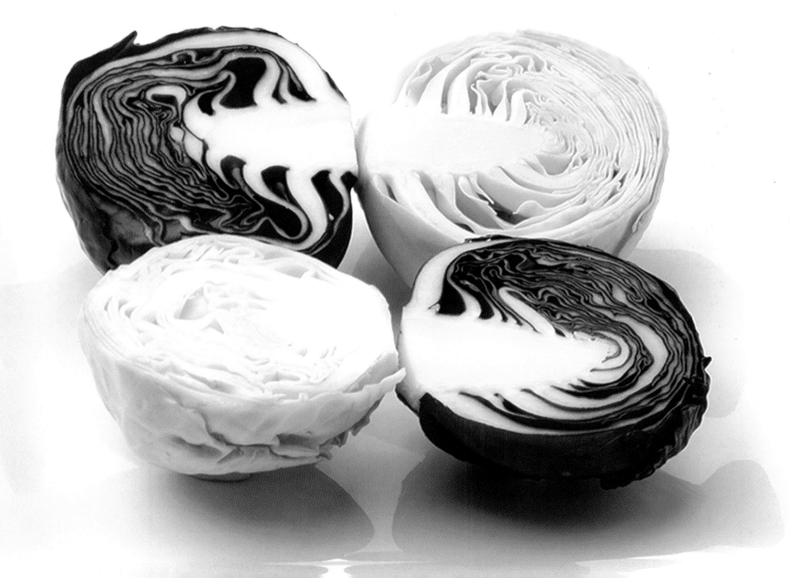

shiitake mushroom

REVERED THROUGH THE CENTURIES FOR THEIR HEALTH-PROMOTING QUALITIES, SHIITAKE MUSHROOMS ARE USED IN THE EAST BOTH TO PREVENT AND TO TREAT DISEASE.

Origins

The shiitake mushroom is a dark, umbrella shaped mushroom with a pungent woody flavour. Its name comes from the Japanese *take*, meaning mushroom, and *shii*, which is the name of the Japanese trees on whose dead wood the mushrooms grow. Native to China and Japan, shiitakes date back many centuries and have come to form a mainstay of the Asian diet. They have long been revered for their medicinal properties, and it is believed that the mushroom was first offered to the Japanese emperor Chaui in the 2nd century CE. Cultivation of the shiitake mushroom is now a growth industry in the US and some parts of Europe owing to its health-giving properties. Shiitakes are widely available in supermarkets and health food shops and can be bought either fresh or dried.

Immune-boosting profile

Shiitake mushrooms have been used to increase resistance to disease for centuries in Traditional Chinese Medicine and they are fast becoming known in the West as a medicinal wonderfood. One particularly remarkable substance in shiitakes, identified by research in Japan, is the immune-boosting phytonutrient lentinan, which has been found to help prevent disease and enhance immune function. Lentinan appears to be able to prevent virus replication and to fight off infection by inducing the production of interferon, the body's own antiviral chemical.

Because of the lentinan it contains, the shiitake has been approved as an official anti-cancer drug in Japan since 1985. Lentinan is used intravenously to increase the survival rate of those with recurrent stomach cancer, by stimulating immune activity. Research also suggests that lentinan may be useful in the fight against AIDS. HIV patients who took concentrated lentinan in liquid form, along with an anti-HIV drug diadanosine, increased their

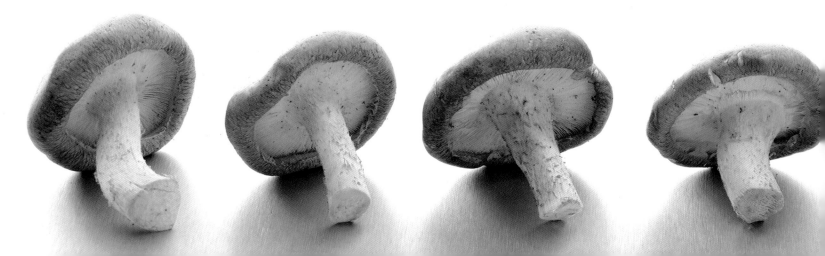

T-cell count for almost three times longer than those patients who took the diadanosine alone. The lentinan in shiitake mushrooms, in combination with conventional drugs, has also been found to help heart-bypass patients fight off infections.

In addition, shiitakes are a useful source of calcium and phosphorus, both important minerals required for forming and maintaining strong bones and teeth. And, as one of the only vegetable sources of vitamin D (which helps the body to retain calcium), they support healthy bones and teeth in children. Shiitakes also contain high levels of certain amino acids including leucine, lysine and threonine. Amino acids are the building blocks of protein, essential for growth and repair. Studies suggest that shiitake mushrooms can also help lower cholesterol and prevent blood clots.

Using shiitake mushrooms in your child's diet

Shiitake mushrooms differ both in taste and texture from ordinary mushrooms. They have a meatier, chewier texture and a stronger, slightly woody, distinctive taste. Some children may find the taste too strong, so it is a good idea to introduce the flavour of shiitake mushrooms mixed with ordinary mushrooms at first.

Shiitake mushrooms are suitable to introduce to your baby at around six months. If you are using fresh shiitake mushrooms, remove the tough stalk, wash the mushroom and chop into small pieces before cooking. This may help to avoid any resistance you might encounter to the new taste. Fresh shiitake mushrooms can replace ordinary mushrooms in soups, stews and mince dishes. They are also delicious in oriental stir-fries and risottos.

If you are using the dried variety of shiitake, you will need to soak them in water for 30 minutes before use. Dried shiitake mushrooms have a much stronger taste than the fresh as they come in a more concentrated form. But, once rehydrated, dried shiitake mushrooms are delicious in a risotto, especially when combined with other mushrooms, such as button, chestnut and oyster.

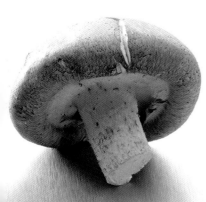

IMMUNE PROFILE

★ B-VITAMINS, VITAMIN D, FOLIC
   ACID; CALCIUM, PHOSPHOROUS

 LENTINAN

✓ ANTICARCINOGENIC, ANTIVIRAL

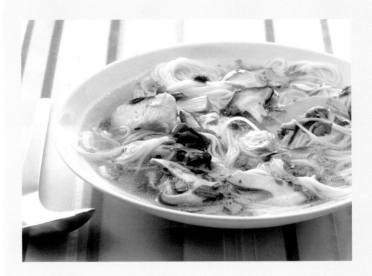

immune booster broth *(above)*

🔆🔆🔆 📋 1⁺ 2⁺ 5⁺

A great recipe for children recovering from illness or for tired teenagers.

A cluster of rice vermicelli noodles
1 tbsp extra virgin olive oil
1 garlic clove, crushed
A handful of shiitake mushrooms, sliced
1 skinless and boneless chicken breast, chopped
600 ml (1 pint) vegetable stock
A slice of fresh ginger
A handful of flat leaf parsley, chopped

Soak the rice vermicelli in a bowl of boiling water for 5 minutes. Meanwhile, heat the olive oil in a pan and add the garlic, shiitake mushrooms and chicken. Cook for a few minutes, stirring all the time. Add the vegetable stock and ginger and simmer gently for 15 minutes. Just before serving add the rice noodles and sprinkle with the parsley.

venison and shiitake casserole

🔆🔆🔆 📋 1⁺ 2⁺ 5⁺

Suitable for all the family, this is delicious served with mashed potato and a green vegetable such as broccoli or green beans.

1 onion, chopped
2 garlic cloves, peeled and crushed
450 g (1 lb) diced venison
10 shiitake mushrooms, washed and sliced
2 large carrots, peeled and chopped
A handful of fresh dates, stoned and chopped
A couple of sprigs of thyme
600 ml (1 pint) vegetable stock
A handful of chopped parsley

Preheat the oven to 190°C/375°F/Gas Mark 5. In a heavy casserole pan, gently cook the onion and garlic in a little olive oil until translucent. Add the meat and brown it well. Add the rest of the ingredients, bring to the boil, cover and transfer to the oven for 1 hour.

KALE

★ BETA-CAROTENE, FOLIC ACID, VITAMINS B3, C AND K; CALCIUM, IRON

▧ CHLOROPHYLL, ISOTHIOCYANATES

✓ ANTICARCINOGENIC, ANTIOXIDANT

Kale is a member of the cabbage family and is a powerhouse of nutrition. It is packed full of vitamin C and beta-carotene, important antioxidants for a healthy immune system. Kale promotes healthy skin and blood clotting and is also rich in iron, which helps protect against anaemia. The calcium content of kale makes it a useful vegetable source of this mineral for children who are vegan or on dairy-free diets. You can now buy baby leaf kale, which many children prefer as its leaves have a softer texture. Add kale to stir-fries or steam it along with other vegetables.

RECIPES: vegetable combos (page 70); cod and veggies (page 73)

SPINACH

★ BETA-CAROTENE, FOLIC ACID, VITAMIN C; IRON, POTASSIUIM

▧ CHLOROPHYLL, LUTEIN

✓ ANTICARCINOGENIC, ANTIOXIDANT

Spinach is rich in the antioxidants vitamin C, beta-carotene and lutein, which help your child's body to fight unstable, disease-causing free radicals and protect it against cancer. Long renowned as an excellent source of iron, spinach, in fact, contains no more iron than any other green leafy vegetable – the confusion was created when scientists calculating its iron content in the 1950s misplaced a decimal point in error! Cooked spinach has a strong, distinctive taste, so raw spinach may be more palatable to many children. If cooked, spinach can be puréed and hidden in stews and pasta dishes. Raw spinach can be simply added to a mixed salad.

RECIPES: vegetable combos (page 70); sardine, anchovy and spinach pâté (page 65); hot salad with balsamic dressing and fresh anchovies (page 98)

OTHER VEGETABLES

BUTTERNUT SQUASH

★ BETA-CAROTENE, VITAMIN E

▧ LUTEIN, ZEAXANTHIN

✓ ANTICARCINOGENIC, ANTIOXIDANT

An extremely popular baby food owing to its sweet, buttery taste, butternut squash is rich in several antioxidant phytonutrients from the carotenoid group. These carotenoids, which give the squash its vivid orange colour, help protect against cancer and boost your child's immune system generally. The beta-carotene in butternut squash is both a potent carotenoid and the plant form of vitamin A, which is needed by your child for healthy skin and vision, as well as for its antioxidant qualities. Antioxidant phytonutrients and antioxidant vitamins work synergystically with each other to further multiply the level of protection that a particular food gives the immune system. Butternut squash can be prepared as a purée, baked in the oven or added to casseroles and soups.

RECIPES: venison steaks with baked butternut squash and cinnamon (page 63); butternut squash and broccoli purée (page 70); vegetable combos (page 70); chicken with butternut squash and coconut (page 96)

PEA

★ FOLIC ACID, VITAMINS B1 AND C

▧ FLAVONOIDS

✓ ANTICARCINOGENIC, ANTIOXIDANT

Owing to their natural sweetness, peas are a popular vegetable with children. Packed full of the antioxidant vitamin C, they help to protect your child against viruses and infection. They also contain folic acid and vitamin B1, both of which keep the nervous system healthy. Peas can be eaten raw straight from the pod or lightly steamed to retain maximum nutritional value.

RECIPES: seafood paella (page 66); venison sausages with pea, mint and potato mash (page 88); vegetable frittata (page 96); queen scallop stir-fry (page 98); immune-boosting chicken broth (page 126)

SWEETCORN

★ BETA-CAROTENE, FOLIC ACID, VITAMIN B3

▧ CURCUMIN, ZEAXANTHIN

✓ ANTICARCINOGENIC, ANTIOXIDANT

Versatile sweetcorn can be eaten straight from the cob or ground into cornmeal, which is a good wheat alternative for allergic children. The vegetable contains plenty of beta-carotene to protect your child's body from disease, as well as curcumin, a phytonutrient with powerful antioxidant and protective properties, which appear to be anti-inflammatory in nature. Sweetcorn is full of fibre, so it is not an ideal first purée for babies as it is hard for an immature system to digest. However, it makes an great finger food for toddlers and older children and is a colourful addition to risottos, pizzas and paellas.

RECIPES: my first fish pie (page 74); quick and easy beany bake (page 80); sweetcorn patties (page 81); family paella (page 98)

fruits

SUMMER FRUITS AND BERRIES

APRICOT

★ BETA-CAROTENE

▨ ANTHOCYANINS, ELLAGIC ACID

✓ ANTICARCINOGENIC, ANTIOXIDANT

Apricots are a rich source of beta-carotene, which your child's body can convert into the vital vitamin A as and when it needs it. This potent antioxidant vitamin protects your child against infection and maintains healthy vision and skin. It also helps to strengthen your child's immune system, so that it can go into rapid attack when it encounters bacteria and viruses. Fresh, juicy apricots are a delicious summer fruit that can be eaten raw (with the stone removed), added to crumbles or pies, or included in Morrocan dishes.

RECIPES: peach and apricot crumble (page 90); 100% fruit jam tarts (page 90)

BLACKBERRY

★ FOLIC ACID, VITAMIN C

▨ ANTHOCYANINS, ELLAGIC ACID

✓ ANTIBACTERIAL, ANTICARCINOGENIC, ANTIOXIDANT

These juicy, dark purple berries are a favourite late-summer fruit. Rich in antibacterial anthocyanins and the antioxidant vitamin C, they help to protect your child against infection at the start of the new school year. Vitamin C also aids iron absorption from other foods and encourages wound healing. Blackberries also contain folic acid, which is vital for a healthy nervous system, and ellagic acid, a phytonutrient that has been found to block the action of cancer-inducing cells. Blackberries are delicious combined with other fruits in crumbles, added to fruit salads or made into jam.

RECIPES: summer fruits compote (page 90)

BLUEBERRY

★ VITAMIN C

▨ ANTHOCYANINS, ELLAGIC ACID

✓ ANTIBACTERIAL, ANTICARCINOGENIC, ANTIOXIDANT

Blueberries are a popular choice with children as they have no pips and are naturally sweet. They contain some vitamin C, which acts as a potent antioxidant. Blueberries are a rich source of anthocyanins, phytonutrients particularly effective at combating E. coli bacteria, which can cause tummy upsets and urinary infections. The fruit also contains the anticancer phytonutrient ellagic acid. They can be eaten raw, or added to pancakes and cooked puddings.

RECIPES: summer fruits brulée (page 66); summer fruits compote (page 90); blueberry smoothie (page 109); hay fever tonic (page 119)

CHERRY

★ VITAMIN C; POTASSIUM

▨ ANTHOCYANINS, ELLAGIC ACID

✓ ANTICARCINOGENIC, ANTIOXIDANT

Cherries are a popular summer fruit and have been used medicinally through the ages for their cleansing and detoxifying properties. They contain some vitamin C but, more importantly, have been identified as a source of the phytonutrients ellagic acid and anthocyanins. Ellagic acid combats cancer-causing cells, and anthocyanins have 20 times the antioxidant power of vitamin C, making them key fighters against harmful free radicals that damage cells and can lead to cancer. Cherries are best eaten fresh and raw. When offering to young children, remember to remove the stones to prevent choking.

RECIPES: nectarine and cherry smoothie (page 99)

CRANBERRY

★ VITAMIN C

▨ ANTHOCYANINS

✓ ANTIBACTERIAL, ANTICARCINOGENIC, ANTIOXIDANT

Because of their intensely sour taste, cranberries are not a suitable berry for the fruit bowl. However, they do have important health-promoting properties as they contain the antioxidant vitamin C, which helps protect your child against infection, and antibacterial substances that can help prevent digestive and urinary infections. Cranberries are best combined with natural sweet flavours or drunk as part of a blend of juices. Commercial cranberry juice drinks often contain large quantities of sugar and are best avoided.

RECIPES: turkey and cranberry burgers (page 79); cranberry and apple smoothie (page 91)

blackcurrant

BLACKCURRANTS ARE A DELICIOUS SUMMER FRUIT SUPERCHARGED WITH A RANGE OF ANTIOXIDANTS THAT PROTECT AND STRENGTHEN YOUR CHILD'S IMMUNE SYSTEM.

Origins

Small and juicy with an intensely sharp taste, blackcurrants have found global popularity for their concentrated health-promoting properties. They come from the *Ribes* family of fruit, which contains three types of currant: the whitecurrant, the blackcurrant and the redcurrant. The gooseberry (*Ribes grossularia*) also belongs to this family. These berries were cultivated in northern Europe before the 17th century and subsequently taken to North America. Following the discovery of vitamin C in the UK in the 1930s, concentrated blackcurrant juice drinks and cordials were commercially produced on a large scale to exploit the country's indigenous source of vitamin C. Subsequently, blackcurrant syrups and lozenges became a popular treatment for relieving the inflammation of sore throats.

Immune-boosting profile

Blackcurrants are packed with a range of antioxidant vitamins and phytonutrients, all of which work together to provide a formidable defence against free radicals (unstable, disease-causing atoms in your child's body). They are a particularly good source of vitamin C. Half a dozen blackcurrants contain more vitamin C than a whole lemon. In fact, other than a guava, there is no other fruit that contains as much vitamin C, weight for weight, as blackcurrants. As an important antioxidant, vitamin C fights free radicals, helping to prevent colds and viral infections, and protects your child's white blood cells from unwanted pathogens (disease-causing microbes). Vitamin C is also essential for the production of antibodies and plays a key role in interferon production. Interferons are proteins that act as antiviral agents, preventing viruses from taking hold in your child's body. They are made and secreted by cells in response to a viral infection and act as messengers to neighbouring cells, telling them that they might be attacked by a virus, and that if they are they must die. In this way, both the cell and the virus contained within it die together.

Blackcurrants are also rich in a group of antioxidant phytonutrients called flavonoids. These help to protect the cells of your child's immune army by deactivating free radicals, which are a by-product of metabolism and can damage cells. Free radicals are usually kept in check by a range of antioxidants found in the diet but their production can be boosted during times of infection or by external factors such as cigarette smoke and pollution. If too many free radicals are produced in the body, they can cause degenerative diseases such as heart disease and cancer. Flavonoids, in partnership with other antioxidants (such as vitamins A, C and E, and zinc and selenium), help combat any increase in free-radical production. Blackcurrants provide an excellent supply

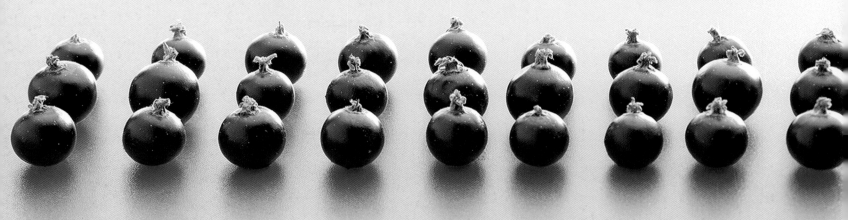

of one group of flavonoids, proanthocyanidins, which have especially potent antioxidant powers, 20 times stronger than those of vitamin C and 50 times the strength of vitamin E. They also reduce inflammation by suppressing histamine release and can be used to fight inflammatory conditions, such as arthritis and allergies. Proanthocyanidins exhibit antibacterial powers, too. In particular, they can inhibit the growth of E. coli, a bacterium that can cause severe stomach upsets and urinary tract infections. E. coli infection is most dangerous in the elderly and children under five, where, in rare cases, it can cause kidney failure.

Blackcurrants are also a source of lutein, one of the group of phytonutrients known as carotenoids that has been identified as having strong antioxidant powers. Like other carotenoids, lutein works synergistically with other antioxidants to provide an increased level of protection. Thus, the combination of antioxidants found in blackcurrants renders them true super-protectors for your child's immune system.

Using blackcurrants in your child's diet

Blackcurrants combine very well with other summer-fruit berries. Because of their tartness, they are often used in sweetened fruit puddings, pies or sauces. They also make excellent jams and jellies and make a lovely addition to a mixed berry smoothie. While there are plenty of recipes with blackcurrants that children will enjoy, it is best to avoid adding refined sugar to sweeten them. Fructose, a slow-releasing fruit sugar that looks similar to caster sugar, is the best alternative sweetener. It tastes sweeter than sugar and can therefore be used in smaller amounts, which is another advantage.

IMMUNE PROFILE

★ VITAMIN C; POTASSIUM

▨ LUTEIN, PROANTHOCYANIDINS

✓ ANTIBACTERIAL, ANTICARCINOGENIC, ANTIHISTAMINE, ANTIOXIDANT

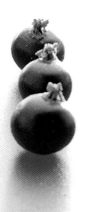

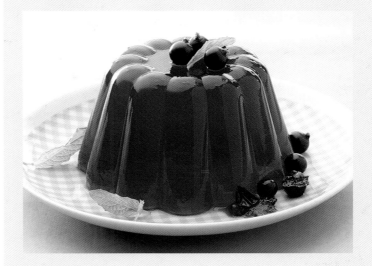

apple and blackcurrant jelly *(above)*

▨▨▨▨ ▨▨▨▨▨   serves 6

This makes a smooth jelly that all children will enjoy. You can buy juice concentrates from health food shops. They contain no added sugar or artificial sweeteners.

½ cup (115 ml/4 fl oz) apple and blackcurrant juice concentrate
2 cups (450 ml/15 fl oz) water
2 sachets of vegegel (or equivalent vegetarian setting agent)

In a saucepan, combine the concentrate with the water and heat until almost boiling. Sprinkle over the vegegel and keep stirring until it has all dissolved. Pour into a jelly mould and allow to cool. Once cooled, place in the fridge until set.

blackcurrant coulis

▨▨▨▨ ▨▨▨▨

This coulis is delicious poured over homemade ice cream or combined with natural yoghurt.

1 cup (150 g/5½ oz) blackcurrants, destalked
½ cup (115 g/4 oz) fructose

Place the blackcurrants in a mixing bowl and cover them with the fructose sugar. Leave for half an hour, then transfer into a food processor and whizz them up. Sieve to create a smooth purée and cool in the fridge before serving.

NECTARINE

★ VITAMIN C

▨ CAROTENOIDS

✓ ANTIOXIDANT

Nectarines are smooth skinned and generally sweeter than their cousins, peaches. For these reasons, they tend to be more popular with children. They are a rich source of vitamin C, an antioxidant and healing vitamin that aids iron absorption and keeps skin healthy. Vitamin C also helps to maintain the efficiency of white blood cells. A great addition to a summer fruit bowl for children to snack on, nectarines can also be blended with other fruits to make smoothies.

RECIPES: *nectarine and cherry smoothie (page 99)*

RED AND BLACK GRAPE

★ POTASSIUM

▨ ANTHOCYANINS, RESERVATOL

✓ ANTICARCINOGENIC, ANTIOXIDANT

Red and black grapes are a good source of phytonutrients called anthocyanins, which are responsible for the fruits' deep rich colour. Research has found these to have immune-boosting antioxidant powers as much as 50 times stronger than vitamin E. Red and black grapes contain reservatol, a phytonutrient that is protective against heart disease, and potassium, which is important for general

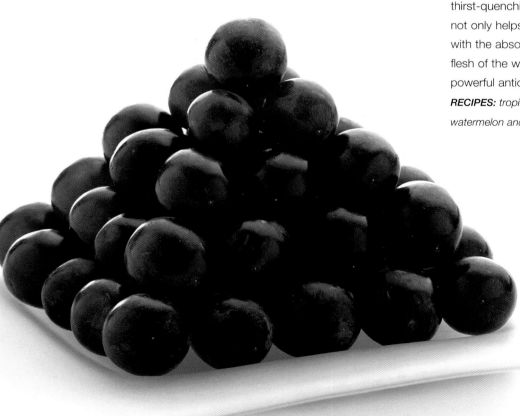

cardiovascular health. Grapes are a great snack food or can be combined with other fruits to make colourful puddings.

RECIPES: *melon, grape and banana smoothie (page 99)*

STRAWBERRY

★ VITAMIN C

▨ ELLAGIC ACID

✓ ANTICARCINOGENIC, ANTIOXIDANT

Strawberries are one of children's favourite summer fruits. Packed full of vitamin C, they strengthen your child's immune defences and protect them from free-radical damage. Strawberries also contain ellagic acid, believed to help prevent cancer. The allergic potential of strawberries is fairly high, so they are best avoided until your child reaches the age of two. They are delicious served plain or mixed with other berries to make puddings and smoothies.

RECIPES: *summer fruits brulée (page 66); strawberry smoothie (page 83); blackcurrant and strawberry ice pops (page 125); protein shake (page 129)*

WATERMELON

★ BETA-CAROTENE, VITAMIN C

▨ LYCOPENE

✓ ANTICARCINOGENIC, ANTIOXIDANT

Watermelon is 95 per cent water, which makes it an excellent thirst-quenching summer snack. The fruit contains vitamin C, which not only helps to protect your child against infection, but also helps with the absorption of iron from other foods. The deep, pinky-red flesh of the watermelon is rich in beta-carotene and lycopene, both powerful antioxidants with additional anti-cancer properties.

RECIPES: *tropical fruit salad with seeds and live yoghurt (page 94); watermelon and ginger ice (page 98)*

EVERYDAY FRUITS

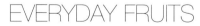

APPLE

★ VITAMIN C; FIBRE

▨ QUERCETIN

✓ ANTI-ALLERGENIC, ANTICARCINOGENIC,
   ANTI-INFLAMMATORY, ANTIOXIDANT

Rich in vitamin C, apples help to strengthen your child's immune defences. The fibre they contain, called pectin, helps to maintain blood sugar levels thereby allowing sustained energy release. Apples also contain quercetin, an antioxidant phytonutrient that also enhances the absorption of vitamin C. In addition, quercetin has antihistamine properties, which makes it a useful anti-allergy substance. Traditionally, apples have been used to treat digestive upsets; offer raw grated apple for constipation and stewed apple for diarrhoea. Apples are a popular and versatile fruit that can be eaten raw or stewed and added to crumbles and pies.

RECIPES: fruit and nut bars (page 66); stewed apple purée with cloves and molasses (page 72); baked apple with raisins and spices (page 75); pheasant paysanne (page 79); breakfast in a glass (page 94); healthy apple strudel (page 99); thyme and chicken casserole (page 107); apple and carrot tonic (page 123); oatbran and berries smoothie (page 131)

BANANA

★ MAGNESIUM, POTASSIUM

✓ AIDS DIGESTION

Bananas are an excellent energy food high in natural sugars that are quickly absorbed into the bloodstream. They are easy to digest and naturally sweet, so make an ideal weaning food for babies. They contain good levels of potassium and magnesium, both calming minerals important for your child's cardiovascular system and for muscle and nerve health. Bananas must be eaten when they are really ripe. This is when the starch in the banana has converted into natural sugars. Unconverted starch in green or unripe bananas can cause tummy aches and constipation. Bananas make an excellent base fruit for a smoothie or homemade ice cream.

RECIPES: porridge with banana, tahini, honey and soaked linseeds (page 62); avocado and banana purée (page 70); fruit smoothie pudding (page 75); banana and raisin cake (page 83); dairy-free ice cream (page 83); kiwi and banana smoothie (page 83); breakfast in a glass (page 94)

LEMON

★ VITAMIN C

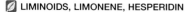 LIMINOIDS, LIMONENE, HESPERIDIN

✓ ANTICARCINOGENIC, ANTIOXIDANT, ANTISEPTIC

Sour tasting, lemons are not a fruit that is often eaten whole. Rather, they are used as a flavouring. The liminoids and limonene found in the pith and rind of the lemon have been recognized to have anticancer effects. Lemon juice is a natural antiseptic and has traditionally been used to soothe sore throats. Rich in vitamin C, lemons can give your child's immune system a useful boost.

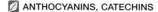 *RECIPES: aioli (page 57); handy hummus with baked potato (page 74); sticky fingers chicken (page 80); healthy apple strudel (page 99); thyme and honey tea (page 107); fresh lemonade (page 119); guacamole (page 119)*

PEAR

★ VITAMIN C; POTASSIUM; FIBRE

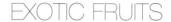 ANTHOCYANINS, CATECHINS

✓ ANTICARCINOGENIC, ANTIOXIDANT

Soft, ripe pears make a popular early weaning food for babies. They are one of the least allergenic foods your child can eat and, with their high water content, they blend well to make a purée. Naturally high in fruit sugars, fibre and the immune-boosting vitamin C, pears should be a fruit bowl staple. They are delicious on their own or added to smoothies or fruit crumbles.

RECIPES: ginger and pear crumble (page 99)

EXOTIC FRUITS

CANTALOUPE MELON

★ BETA-CAROTENE, VITAMIN C

▨ CAROTENOIDS

✓ ANTICARCINOGENIC, ANTIOXIDANT

Cantaloupe melons are a sweet, tropical fruit popular with children. Unlike the other varieties of melon, they contain beta-carotene, an antioxidant that your child's body can convert into vitamin A. They are also a good source of vitamin C, which protects your child from infection. Serve raw, or in a fresh juice or smoothie.

RECIPES: tropical fruit salad with seeds and live yoghurt (page 94); melon, grape and banana smoothie (page 99); hay fever tonic (page 119)

GUAVA

★ VITAMIN C; POTASSIUM

▨ LYCOPENE

✓ ANTICARCINOGENIC, ANTIOXIDANT

Guavas originate from South America and contain more vitamin C, weight for weight, than any other fruit. Vitamin C is a powerful antioxidant that helps to strengthen your child's immune system by fighting disease-causing free radicals. For children, guavas can be peeled and deseeded and the flesh eaten plain, blended in a smoothie or combined with other tropical fruits in a fruit salad.

RECIPES: guava smoothie (page 117)

KIWI FRUIT

★ VITAMIN C; POTASSIUM

▨ CHLOROPHYLL

✓ ANTICARCINOGENIC, ANTIOXIDANT

Kiwi fruit contains chlorophyll, which not only gives the fruit its green colouring but has also been found to inhibit the growth of cancerous cells. Kiwi fruit is a rich source of vitamin C, and of potassium which is good for heart, muscle and nerve health. The vivid green and black colours make kiwi an eye-catching addition to fruit salads, and blended with banana it makes a great antioxidant-rich smoothie.

RECIPES: kiwi and banana smoothie (page 83); tropical fruit salad with seeds and live yoghurt (page 94); hay fever tonic (page 119)

MANGO

★ BETA-CAROTENE, VITAMIN C; FIBRE

▨ CRYPTOXANTHIN AND OTHER CAROTENOIDS

✓ ANTICARCINOGENIC, ANTIOXIDANT

Mangoes are rich in the antioxidants beta-carotene and vitamin C, which boost your child's immune defences and provide protection against cell damage and disease. They are also a good source of insoluble fibre, which has a cleansing action on the bowel. Mangoes contain cryptoxanthin, which may help to reduce the risk of certain cancers. Naturally sweet, mangoes are popular with children and are delicious eaten raw or mixed with Indian or other Eastern dishes.

RECIPES: mint and mango smoothie (page 66); mango hedgehog (page 83); pineapple and mango jelly (page 91); hay fever tonic (page 119)

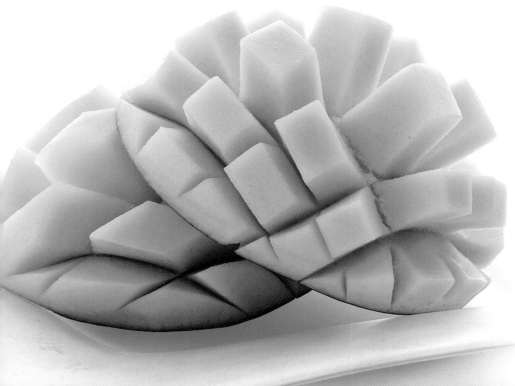

PAPAYA (PAW PAW)

★ BETA-CAROTENE, VITAMINS C AND E

▨ CRYPTOXANTHIN AND OTHER CAROTENOIDS

✓ ANTICARCINOGENIC, ANTIOXIDANT

The papaya is an antioxidant powerhouse packed with immune-boosting vitamins and phytonutrients, which help your child's body to neutralize potentially damaging free radicals and maintain immunity. Its antioxidant content includes the carotenoids, which provide the fruit's orange colouring, and vitamins C and E, which are also needed for skin and mucous membrane health. Papayas are known for helping to eliminate mucus from the body, so are good at providing relief for the many coughs and colds of childhood. They are delicious combined with natural yoghurt or added to fruit salads.

RECIPES: four fruit purée (page 51); papaya and lime smoothie (page 91); tropical fruit salad with seeds and live yoghurt (page 94)

PINEAPPLE

★ VITAMIN C

▨ BROMELAIN

✓ AIDS DIGESTION, ANTI-INFLAMMATORY, ANTIOXIDANT

Pineapples are rich in vitamin C and in the plant enzyme bromelain. Vitamin C aids wound healing and iron absorption, and is good for general skin health. It also has powerful immune-boosting antioxidant properties. Bromelain has been much studied for its potential healing powers and has been used therapeutically for arthritis, owing to its anti-inflammatory nature. The enzyme also helps to break down protein in the body, thereby aiding digestion.

RECIPES: tropical smoothie (page 35); pineapple and mango jelly (page 91); sweet and sour prawn stir-fry with egg noodles and bok choi (page 96)

PINK GRAPEFRUIT

★ BETA-CAROTENE, VITAMIN C

▨ LYCOPENE, HESPERIDIN

✓ ANTICARCINOGENIC, ANTIOXIDANT

Pink grapefruit is a sweeter variety of grapefruit than the plain yellow. The fruit is also a richer source of vitamin C and its pink pigment contains beta-carotene and the phytonutrient lycopene. Research suggests that lycopene's antioxidant powers can prevent certain forms of cancer. Some children love the flavour of grapefruit, so try it in a fruit salad or a delicious smoothie.

DRIED FRUITS

DATE

★ B-VITAMINS; IRON, MAGNESIUM, POTASSIUM

✓ NATURAL SWEETENER

! RISK OF DENTAL CARIES

Dates are a wonderful alternative sweetener to sugar and make an excellent purée to combine with cereals for babies. They are rich in potassium and magnesium, which are important for muscles, nerves and the development and maintenance of healthy bones and teeth. As they are such a concentrated source of fruit sugar, dates should not be used as an everyday snack.

RECIPES: *date purée (page 72)*

DRIED APRICOT

★ IRON, POTASSIUM

▨ BROMELAIN

✓ ANTIANAEMIC

! RISK OF DENTAL CARIES

Dried apricots are a good source of iron, which helps the blood carry oxygen to all parts of the body. Without sufficient iron, your child will feel tired and be more susceptible to infection. Dried apricots that are bright orange have been treated with sulphur dioxide (E220), which can cause allergic reactions and is therefore best avoided. Unsulphured dried apricots are dark in colour and are available in health food shops. They make a delicious purée for babies and a popular snack for older children.

RECIPES: *semolina fruit pudding with dried apricot purée (page 75)*

RAISIN

★ IRON, POTASSIUM

✓ ANTIANAEMIC, NATURAL SWEETENER

! RISK OF DENTAL CARIES

Raisins are popular with children and are a good source of iron. They make a great natural sweetener in baking but are a concentrated form of fruit sugar, so it is better to offer them at mealtimes or combined with other foods to prevent dental caries.

RECIPES: *baked apple with raisins and spices (page 75); banana and raisin cake (page 83); healthy apple strudel (page 99)*

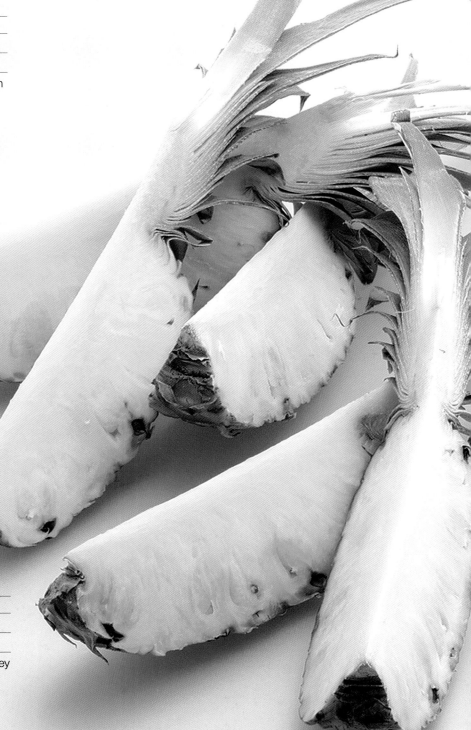

orange

ORANGES PROVIDE HIGH LEVELS OF ANTIOXIDANT VITAMINS AND PHYTONUTRIENTS TO BATTLE VIRAL INFECTION AND KEEP YOUR CHILD'S IMMUNE SYSTEM IN OPTIMUM HEALTH.

Origins

Oranges are part of the citrus family (*Rutacaceae*), which also includes lemons, limes, grapefruits, tangerines and clementines. There are many different varieties of orange – some bitter and some sweet – such as the navel orange, the blood orange, the mandarin, the Jaffa orange and the Seville orange. The navel orange is seedless and sweet and has a thick skin that is easy to peel. The blood orange, also sweet, has ruby-red flesh and can be either juiced or eaten peeled. The mandarin is similar to a tangerine. Jaffa oranges can be sharper in taste and are often used for juicing. The Seville orange is sour and traditionally used for making marmalade.

The word orange is derived from the fruit's Sanskrit name, *naranga*, which means fragrant. Oranges originated in China and were used initially for the fragrance of their rind. Once cultivated in China and India, they moved westwards to Arabia and from there to the countries surrounding the Mediterranean coast. The first oranges to appear in Europe were recorded as early as the 13th century. These were bitter oranges and sweet varieties did not arrive until the later part of the 15th century. Christopher Columbus took orange and other citrus plant seeds to the New World on his second voyage in 1493. Oranges are now cultivated worldwide but grow best in hot countries with a sub-tropical climate.

Immune-boosting profile

Oranges are probably best known for their vitamin C content. Vitamin C helps to protect your child's body from infection. It strengthens the immune army and, as a powerful antioxidant, it neutralizes harmful free radicals, thereby potentially inhibiting the development of certain degenerative diseases such as cancer. Vitamin C also plays a key role in the production of collagen, a substance in the skin that is a critical factor in wound healing. One further advantage of vitamin C is that it aids the body's absorption of iron from other foods. This is particularly relevant for children and teenagers, who often have low iron stores. Iron is vital for growing children and a lack of it can result in the deficiency disease anaemia, which can cause poor physical development and learning difficulties. Eating an orange or drinking orange juice with a meal will maximize the absorption of iron from the foods eaten.

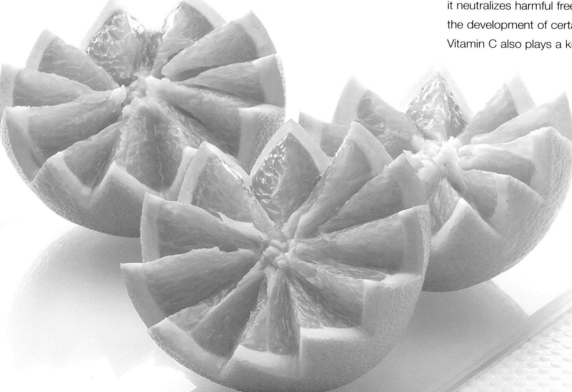

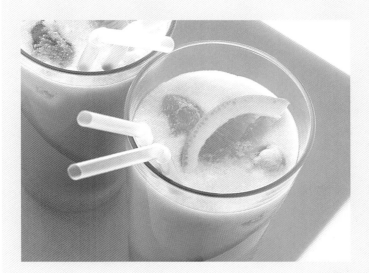

In common with other citrus fruits, oranges contain more than 100 different phytonutrients that are beneficial to health. They are a very good source of flavonoids, the antioxidant phytonutrients that act synergistically with vitamin C to boost your child's protection against free-radical damage. Hesperidin is an important known flavonoid found in oranges, which has additional antiviral, anti-allergenic and anti-inflammatory properties. Oranges and other citrus fruits also contain the phytonutrient limonene, which is thought to have anticarcinogenic properties. All oranges contain the carotenoid phytonutrients beta-carotene, beta-cryptoxanthin and zeaxanthin. These carotenoids have potent antioxidant powers that boost the immune system and help protect your child from disease.

Using oranges in your child's diet

While oranges are enormously beneficial to health, whether you eat the whole fruit or just drink the delicious juice, it is worth noting that the whole fruit contains many more nutrients than pure orange juice alone. Most of an orange's flavonoids are found in the pith and rind of the fruit, as is its fibre, pectin, which protects your child's cardiovascular system with its cholesterol-lowering abilities.

As they have to travel huge distances from harvesting to the fruit bowl, most oranges are waxed and coloured to extend their shelf life and protect their appearance. If you are using the rind of an orange in a recipe, use an unwaxed fruit. The wax, which contains fungicides, has been associated with a higher risk of cancer. You can tell if an orange has been waxed as it will be very shiny and you will be able to scrape off the wax with your fingernail.

Oranges can cause allergic reactions in susceptible children and adults, triggering a migraine or causing skin rashes. For this reason, I do not recommend giving orange or orange juice to your baby until she reaches the age of one.

Oranges make delicious fresh juices either alone or combined with other fruits. Always dilute fresh fruit juices with water for small children, as the juice is naturally sweet and can be too acidic for baby teeth. Other easily peeled citrus fruit varieties, such as clementines and tangerines, make great additions to lunch boxes and picnics.

IMMUNE PROFILE

★ BETA-CAROTENE, FOLIC ACID, VITAMIN C; FIBRE

▨ BETA-CRYPTOXANTHIN, HESPERIDIN, LIMONENE, ZEAXANTHIN

✓ ANTI-ALLERGENIC, ANTICARCINOGENIC, ANTI-INFLAMMATORY,
  ANTIOXIDANT, ANTIVIRAL

orange surprise *(above)*

serves 2

Juice of 4 oranges
Juice of ½ lime
Zest of ½ unwaxed lime
A little grated ginger
1 banana
A handful of crushed ice cubes

In a liquidizer, blend all the ingredients together and serve immediately.

carrot and orange soup

serves 2

1 onion, finely chopped
1 tbsp extra virgin olive oil
4 large carrots, peeled and chopped
Grated rind of ½ an orange
600 ml (1 pint) vegetable stock
Juice of 2 oranges
1 tbsp chopped coriander

In a saucepan, gently cook the onion in the oil until translucent. Add the carrots, orange rind and the stock and simmer for 20 minutes. Liquidize the soup with the orange juice. Sprinkle with the coriander to serve.

tropical smoothie

Juice of 2 oranges
1 small pineapple, peeled and decored
2 ripe bananas
1 cup of coconut milk
1 tbsp linseed oil

Put all the ingredients into a liquidizer and blend until smooth.

nuts and seeds

ALMOND

★ B-VITAMINS, VITAMIN E; CALCIUM, MAGNESIUM

▨ PHYTIC ACID

✓ ANTIOXIDANT, BONE BUILDING, HIGH ENERGY FOOD

Almonds are rich in the antioxidant vitamin E, which boosts your child's immune system. They are a good source of calcium, which is not only required for healthy bones and teeth, but also plays an important part in immune function. Essential fatty acid metabolism is dependant on the presence of calcium, among other nutrients, and essential fats help regulate the immune system and keep it working at full capacity. Almonds have a low allergic potential and so are an ideal first nut to be introduced to a child. Give only ground almonds to a child under five because of the potential choking hazard.

RECIPES: *almond lassi (page 51); ginger cake (page 66); my first muesli (page 72); nut butter sandwiches (page 86); chicken and almond satay with carrot and sesame stir-fry (page 88); peach and apricot crumble (page 90)*

CASHEW NUT

★ B-VITAMINS, FOLIC ACID; IRON, MAGNESIUM, SELENIUM, ZINC

✓ ANTICARCINOGENIC, ANTIOXIDANT

Cashews contain many important nutrients for your child's immune system. Iron, zinc and B-vitamins are all required for the production of important cells in the immune army, and selenium plays a key role in protection against cancer. In addition, the minerals found in cashews are important for essential fatty acid metabolism, another vital function for immune health. With their creamy texture, cashew nuts make an ideal addition to smoothies and ice creams.

RECIPES: *roasted vegetables with coriander couscous (page 65); creamy cashew porridge (page 78); carrot and cashew nut soup (page 80); dairy-free ice cream (page 83); nut butter sandwiches (page 86)*

LINSEED

★ MAGNESIUM; FIBRE, OMEGA-3 ESSENTAIL FATTY ACIDS

▨ LIGNANS

✓ ANTICARCINOGENIC, ANTI-INFLAMMATORY, ANTIOXIDANT

Linseeds are a wonderful source of omega-3 essential fatty acids, which are necessary for the proper regulation of the immune army.

They are also a good source of fibre, which helps to keep bowel movements regular. Linseeds contain lignans, a group of phytonutrients that have been found to have anti-cancer properties. Linseeds are found in concentrated form in linseed oil (flaxseed oil). This tends to be the most convenient way to supply your child with enough of the important essential fatty acids contained in the linseeds. Linseed oil can be added to smoothies and dressings without detection! It is, however, an unstable oil that should not be used for cooking at heat and should be kept in the fridge to prevent it from going rancid.

RECIPES: *porridge with banana, tahini, honey and soaked linseeds (page 62); my first muesli (page 72); strawberry smoothie (page 83); crunchy muesli (page 86); breakfast in a glass (page 94); garlic and honey dressing (page 117)*

PINE NUT

★ VITAMIN E; IRON, MAGNESIUM, POTASSIUM, ZINC

✓ ANTICARCINOGENIC, ANTIOXIDANT

Pine nuts are the seeds of the pine tree and have recently found international popularity. They provide an excellent source of polyunsaturated fats and the antioxidant vitamin E, which supports the immune system and is important for cell membrane health. Pine nuts are also a source of the immune-boosting minerals zinc and iron. They are delicious as part of a salad and are an important ingredient in the popular Italian pasta sauce, pesto.

RECIPES: *nutty pesto (page 39); walnut bread (page 63); pine nut, avocado, red onion and watercress salad sandwich (page 65); fresh tomato, avocado and pine nut pasta sauce with balsamic vinegar (page 97)*

PUMPKIN SEED

★ FOLIC ACID, VITAMIN E; IRON, MAGNESIUM, ZINC

▨ PHYTOSTEROLS

✓ ANTICARCINOGENIC, ANTIOXIDANT

Zinc has many nutritional benefits for your child, such as helping to ensure healthy mental and physical development. As pumpkin seeds contain the highest levels of zinc of all the seed types, they are an excellent seed to introduce to your children early on. Zinc is also required for more than 200 enzymatic processes in your child's body. It helps to keep your child's thymus in good shape as well as protecting against infection. Pumpkin seeds also contain phytosterols, phytonutrients with anticarcinogenic qualities. In common with other edible seeds, pumpkin seeds can be ground and added to porridge and other cereals, roasted and added to salads, or combined with other nuts and seeds to make muesli bars.

RECIPES: roasted vegetables with coriander couscous (page 65); family salads (page 81); crunchy muesli (page 86); breakfast in a glass (page 94)

SESAME SEED AND TAHINI

★ VITAMINS B3 AND E; CALCIUM, MAGNESIUM, ZINC; FIBRE

▨ PHYTIC ACID, SESAMINOL

✓ ANTICARCINOGENIC, ANTIOXIDANT

Sesame seeds and tahini (pulped sesame seeds) are packed full of nutrients for your child's immune system. They are a rich source of calcium and magnesium and, as such, are a particularly useful source of these minerals for children with dairy allergies. Sesame seeds have substantial antioxidant strength due to the vitamin E, sesaminol and phytic acid that they contain. Phytic acid has been shown to inhibit the growth of cancer cells. Sesame seeds can be added to biscuits and muesli bars; tahini can be added to baby purées or soups, and is a key ingredient in tasty hummus.

RECIPES: porridge with banana, tahini, honey and soaked linseeds (page 62); sesame pitta strips (page 63); handy hummus with baked potato (page 74); sweet potato and tahini (page 74); muesli squares (page 83); chicken and almond satay with carrot and sesame stir-fry (page 88); sesame and honey bars (page 99)

SPROUTED SEEDS

★ B-VITAMINS, FOLIC ACID, VITAMIN C

▨ CAROTENOIDS, COUMESTROL, SAPONINS

✓ ANTICARCINOGENIC, ANTIOXIDANT

Along with sprouted beans, sprouted seeds are a wonderful source of vitamins and phytonutrients. The best-known sprouted seeds and beans are alfalfa, mung beansprouts and soya beansprouts. By sprouting you enhance their nutritional value. Sprouting seeds is cheap and easy and something your children will really enjoy doing. Simply take a handful of the seeds or beans, rinse well and soak in tepid water for 12 hours. Drain, rinse and put in a lidded container. Rinse and drain well twice a day, returning them to the container in between. In two to six days,

depending on the seed or bean used, you should have your sprouted seeds. Place in a sealed bag. They will keep in the fridge for up to a week. Alfalfa, mung and soya beansprouts contain coumestrol, a phytonutrient that displays antioxidant, anti-inflammatory and anticarcinogenic abilities. Sprouts can be added to salads and sandwiches or combined in a raw baby purée.

RECIPES: family salads (page 81); energy salad with garlic and honey dressing (page 117)

SUNFLOWER SEED

★ B-VITAMINS, VITAMIN E; IRON, MAGNESIUM, MANGANESE; ESSENTIAL FATTY ACIDS

▨ LIGNANS

✓ ANTICARCINOGENIC, ANTI-INFLAMMATORY, ANTIOXIDANT

Sunflower seeds are rich in the nutrients needed to support a healthy immune system. They contain the antioxidant vitamin E, which helps to protect your child from infection, and are a good source of essential fatty acids (EFAs), which keep your child's skin healthy as well as regulating the activities of their immune army. Sunflower seeds make an excellent snack food; they can also be added to breads and biscuits or sprinkled on salads.

RECIPES: roasted vegetables with coriander couscous (page 65); family salads (page 81); crunchy muesli (page 86); energy salad with garlic and honey dressing (page 117)

walnut

WALNUTS ARE EXCELLENT SOURCES OF ANTIOXIDANT NUTRIENTS AND PROVIDE HIGH LEVELS OF ESSENTIAL FATTY ACIDS, WHICH ARE REQUIRED FOR OPTIMUM BRAIN FUNCTION AND THE REGULATION OF A HEALTHY IMMUNE SYSTEM.

Origins

Walnuts are part of the tree nut family, which also includes pecan nuts. There are around 20 species of walnut, but the best-known are the Persian walnut (*Juglans regia*), sometimes called the English walnut, and the black walnut (*Juglans nigra*). The Persian walnut is the most popular and has a smooth, tan-coloured shell that is easy to crack. The black walnut, which is native to North America, has a stronger flavour and is covered by a very rough shell that is hard to crack. The Persian walnut was sent from Persia to Ancient Greece and made its way through Europe during Roman times. It finally arrived in Britain in the 15th century. Walnut oil was a highly prized cooking ingredient in the Middle Ages and it is enjoying something of a renaissance in cooking today.

Immune-boosting profile

Walnuts are rich in vitamin E and selenium. Along with vitamin C and beta-carotene, these nutrients are particularly good antioxidants, which help protect your child against illness by keeping disease-promoting free radicals in check. Vitamin E is also required for healthy skin and wound healing, both important in the growing child. Selenium, which is needed for essential hormone production and for growth and fertility, works alongside vitamin E to multiply their combined antioxidant action.

Walnuts also contain high levels of ellagic acid, a phytonutrient that has anticarcinogenic effects and antioxidant powers. Ellagic acid belongs to the large group of phytonutrients known as phenolic compounds. These compounds also exhibit antibacterial, anti-inflammatory and antithrombotic effects.

Perhaps the key nutritional benefit of walnuts is found in their rich essential fatty acid (EFA) content. These fats, which are vital for a child's development and for the proper functioning of the immune system, are essential because they can only be obtained directly through diet. There are two families of EFAs. The omega-6 family is found in foods such as safflower oil, sunflower oil, evening primrose oil and corn oil. The omega-3 family of EFAs, which is found in walnuts and walnut oil, is also found in food-grade linseed (flaxseed) oil, soyabean and wheatgerm oil, and in fresh oily fish such as mackerel, tuna, herring and salmon. These families of EFAs play a key role in your child's immune system. In the presence of vitamins A, B6, C and E, as well as the minerals zinc,

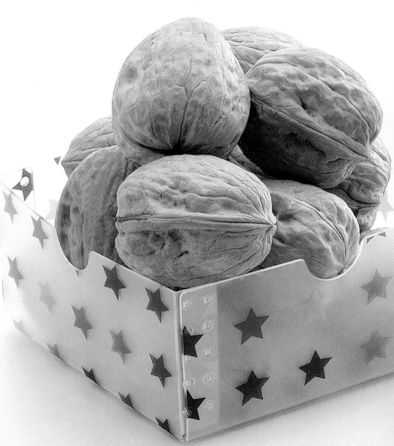

magnesium, calcium, copper and selenium, they are converted into chemical messengers called prostaglandins, which perform many functions including regulating the activity of the white blood cells, part of your child's immune army. Without sufficient EFAs in her diet, your child's immune system is not functioning at full capacity and this will make her more susceptible to colds, infections and allergies. Prostaglandins formed from omega-6 EFAs also help to maintain blood sugar levels, prevent blood clots by thinning the blood and act as anti-inflammatory agents bringing pain relief to conditions such as arthritis. The omega-3 fats convert into prostaglandins that are crucial for proper brain function, which includes coordination, memory, learning ability, mood and vision.

Sadly, children's diets today are frequently lacking in the seeds, oils and fish that can supply the essential fats they need to produce these prostaglandins. Furthermore, their diets are laden with sugar and damaged fats found in fast foods and processed foods that interfere with the basic steps of essential fatty acid metabolism.

Using walnuts in your child's diet

The novelty of cracking open fresh walnuts and prising them out of their shells provides great entertainment value for children and is a good way to introduce them to the taste of fresh nuts. Shelled and chopped walnuts should be bought vacuum-packed and stored in an airtight container in the fridge as they tend to become rancid more quickly than fresh nuts. Walnuts, like other nuts, should not be introduced to your baby before nine months and at this age nuts should always be ground. To guard against choking, it is best to wait until the age of five before giving whole walnuts to children.

Walnuts make a great addition to salads, rice dishes, puddings and cake decorations. They can also be easily disguised, as in the case of walnut biscuits (see right). Using walnut oil is another crafty means of incorporating walnuts into your child's diet. Mixed in dressings and added to baking dishes, it brings flavour as well as excellent health benefits. However, walnut oil is relatively unstable and should never be used for frying food at a high heat.

IMMUNE PROFILE

★ VITAMIN E; POTASSIUM, SELENIUM; OMEGA-3 EFAS

▨ ELLAGIC ACID, FLAVONOIDS

✓ ANTI-ALLERGENIC, ANTIBACTERIAL, ANTICARCINOGENIC,
ANTI-INFLAMMATORY, ANTIOXIDANT

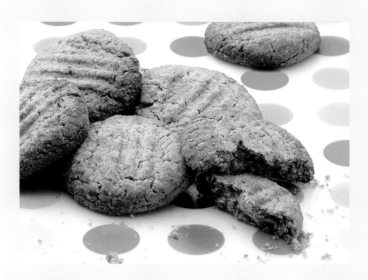

walnut biscuits *(above)*

▨▨▨▨ ▨ 1+ 2+ 5+   Makes 12–15 biscuits

These delicious biscuits are an ideal way of introducing walnuts into your child's diet.

1½ cups (175 g/6 oz) self-raising wholemeal flour
½ cup (175 g/ 6 oz) runny honey (warmed)
½ cup (115 ml/4 fl oz) walnut oil
½ cup (60 g/2 oz) ground walnuts

Preheat the oven to 200°C/400°F/Gas Mark 6. Place all the ingredients in a large bowl and mix well to form a dough. Next, form small balls out of the mixture and place them on a baking tray. Flatten them gently with a fork. Bake for 8 minutes. Leave to cool on a wire rack and store in an airtight container.

nutty pesto

▨▨▨▨ ▨ 1+ 2+ 5+

Rich in essential fatty acids, protein and antioxidants, this pesto contains plenty of immune-boosting power.

2 tbsp walnuts
2 tbsp pine nuts
¼ cup (40 g/1½ oz) grated parmesan cheese
½ cup (25 g/1 oz) fresh basil
2 garlic cloves
½ cup (115 ml/4 fl oz) extra virgin olive oil

Whizz all the ingredients together in a food processor to make a smooth paste. If too thick, add a little more olive oil until you reach the desired consistency.

grains

AMARANTH

★ CALCIUM, MAGNESIUM; LYSINE

✓ ANTIVIRAL

Amaranth is an ancient Aztec grain that has recently become known internationally. It is rich in amino acids, notably lysine, which can help to protect your child against the herpes family of viruses (see glandular fever, pages 116–17). Amaranth can be cooked and served in the same way as rice or popped like popcorn.

BARLEY

★ B-VITAMINS, FOLIC ACID, VITAMIN E; MAGNESIUM

 PROTEASE INHIBITORS

✓ ANTICARCINOGENIC, ANTIOXIDANT, ANTIVIRAL

Whole barley or pot barley is more nutritious than pearl barley, which is a refined grain that has had most of its nutrients stripped out during the refining process. Barley does contain gluten and is therefore not suitable for any child on a gluten-free diet, such as a sufferer of coeliac disease. However, it also contains phytonutrients called protease inhibitors that have anti-cancer effects. In addition, barley has antioxidant and antiviral properties, and has traditionally been used to treat digestive complaints and urinary infections. Barley makes a great addition to soups and stews.

RECIPES: *braised broth of guinea fowl with winter vegetables (page 47); immunity soup (page 123)*

BROWN RICE

★ B-VITAMINS; CALCIUM, IRON; FIBRE

 PHYTIC ACID

✓ ANTICARCINOGENIC, EASILY DIGESTED

Rice is a gluten-free grain that makes an excellent early food for babies. Brown rice contains all the nutrients that white rice has had removed during the refining process. Rice has traditionally been used to treat digestive complaints and brown rice is a good remedy for constipation. Rice milk is an excellent convalescent drink especially when dairy products need to be avoided, as in the case of gastroenteritis, for example. Brown rice contains phytic acid, a phytonutrient that exhibits anticarcinogenic properties. Add

brown rice to soups, include it in risottos and paellas or use ground brown rice flakes to make porridge for a baby.

RECIPES: *seafood paella (page 66); family paella (page 98); salmon and broccoli risotto (page 103); salmon kedgeree (page 113)*

BUCKWHEAT

★ VITAMIN A; CALCIUM, SELENIUM

 RUTIN

✓ ANTIOXIDANT

Buckwheat is the staple grain in Russia and Poland. It is not, as its name suggests, related to wheat. It is an antioxidant, gluten-free grain, and is a rich source of rutin, a phytonutrient that helps strengthen your child's blood vessels. Buckwheat should be bought ready-roasted and can be added to soups and stews or used to make pilaffs. The flour can be used to make delicious pancakes.

RECIPES: *my first pasta sauce (page 73); tempting tofu pasta sauce (page 74)*

MILLET

★ SILICON; FIBRE

 ISOFLAVONES

✓ ALKALINE, ANTICARCINOGENIC, EASILY DIGESTED

Millet is an alkaline gluten-free grain, which makes an excellent first cereal for a baby as it is both gentle on the stomach and has very low allergic potential. It is a good source of protein and contains anticarcinogenic phytonutrients. Millet is rich in silicon, a mineral needed for healthy skin, hair, teeth, eyes and nails. It can be prepared as a porridge using millet flakes or boiled like rice in the grain form.

RECIPES: *millet porridge with date purée (page 72)*

POPCORN

★ BETA-CAROTENE, VITAMIN E; MAGNESIUM, POTASSIUM

✓ ANTI-ALLERGENIC, ANTICARCINOGENIC, ANTIOXIDANT

This gluten-free grain makes an excellent snack food for children, as it is free from salt, sugar and other unwanted additives. It is also a useful addition to the diet of a child who has a wheat allergy. Introduce after the age of one to avoid the risk of choking.

RECIPES: *popcorn (page 90)*

QUINOA

★ B-VITAMINS, VITAMIN E; CALCIUM, IRON

 SAPONINS

✓ ANTICARCINOGENIC, ANTIOXIDANT

Quinoa is a South American grain that contains more calcium than milk and has the highest level of protein out of all the grains. For this reason, it is an excellent grain to incorporate in a vegetarian or vegan diet. Quinoa must be washed well before cooking to remove its bitter coating. It can be mixed with other grains to make porridge, added to soups and stews or served as an accompaniment instead of rice.

RECIPES: shiitake, spring onion and bok choi stir-fry with quinoa (page 111)

WHEATGERM

★ B-VITAMINS, VITAMIN E; IRON

✓ ANTICARCINOGENIC, ANTIOXIDANT

Wheatgerm is the product left behind after the processing of refined flour. It is, therefore, the best bit, containing all the nutrients that have been stripped from the finished product. Rich in both the antioxidant vitamin E and iron, wheatgerm is a great addition to the diet of any wheat- and gluten-tolerant child. Add it to smoothies, sprinkle on cereals and yoghurt or combine with oats to make a tasty crumble.

RECIPES: protein shake (page 62); breakfast in a glass (page 94); ginger and pear crumble (page 99)

WHOLEWHEAT

★ B-VITAMINS, VITAMIN E; IRON; FIBRE

 LIGNANS

✓ ANTICARCINOGENIC, ANTIOXIDANT

Recent research indicates that up to a third of cancers could be prevented by eating three portions of wholegrains a day. Wholegrains are products derived from the unrefined whole grain of a cereal crop, in the case of wholewheat, from wheat. Wholemeal flour, used for making wholemeal bread and pasta among other things, is a form of wholewheat. Wholewheat is rich in B-vitamins as well as the antioxidant vitamin E. It also helps prevent constipation, a common problem in children on a refined diet. Wheat products are a common source of allergy and intolerance among children, so incorporating other types of wholegrains, such as brown rice, millet, buckwheat, oats, quinoa and corn, into their diet is beneficial.

RECIPES: quick and easy seafood pasta supper (page 63); fruity scotch pancakes (page 78); muesli squares (page 83); nut butter sandwiches (page 86); homemade soda bread (page 95); ginger and pear crumble (page 99)

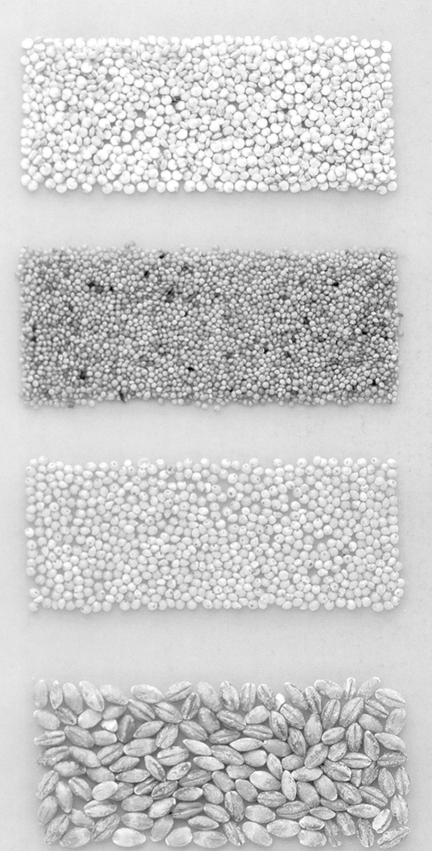

oats

OATS ARE A POPULAR AND VERSATILE GRAIN, PACKED FULL OF ANTIOXIDANTS AND A HOST OF OTHER NUTRIENTS THAT SUPPORT YOUR CHILD'S IMMUNE SYSTEM THROUGH TO ADULTHOOD.

Origins

The cultivation of wild oats (*Avena sativa*) can be traced back to around 1000BCE. Neither the Greeks nor the Romans liked to eat oats themselves, and at the time they were used mostly as animal feed. Oats were considered a hardy crop that could grow even in the most unwelcome soil and the Romans spread their cultivation to Britain, where they quickly became a staple part of the diet. The cultivation of oats in America began in the 17th century and, today, North America, Europe and the countries of the former Soviet Union grow 90 per cent of the world's oat crops.

Immune-boosting profile

Oats are among the most nutritious grains you can give to your child. Carbohydrate makes up the greater part of the grain as with other grains, but oats have a higher level of protein (between 15 and 20 per cent) than other grains and offer one other significant advantage – they also contain good levels of polyunsaturated fats. These fats include linoleic acid, part of the omega-6 essential fatty acid family, which helps support a strong immune system and healthy blood.

Oats have received much attention in the last few years for their ability to maintain blood sugar levels. This is because they are slow-releasing carbohydrates, rich in protein and a certain type of fibre called beta-glucan, which slow the body's rate of glucose conversion allowing sustainable energy release. After a meal, your child's body digests the food eaten and converts it into glucose, the only type of fuel it can use to create energy. Glucose enters the bloodstream and is carried around the body refuelling the cells. If your child's diet is full of sugary foods and drinks and refined carbohydrates, such as white flour, white sugar and white rice, the conversion of food to glucose happens rapidly, causing too much glucose to enter the bloodstream at once. The body reacts by releasing insulin, a hormone that lowers the glucose levels in the blood (blood sugar) by dispersing it to cells and converting any excess into fat that can be stored in the child's body. In a child with a poor diet, this chemical reaction can happen several times a day, resulting in blood sugar levels that bounce up and down causing symptoms such as tiredness, irritability, moodiness, aggression and tearfulness.

Oats are also rich in the antioxidants vitamin E and zinc, which protect your child from free-radical damage. Both zinc and vitamin E help to maintain the body's thymus gland (see page 12) and aid essential fatty acid metabolism. Vitamin E also protects the fat in the oats, which helps prevent rancidity, and zinc is required by the body for the production of white blood cells.

Other immune-boosting vitamins and minerals found in high levels in oats include B-vitamins, calcium, magnesium and iron. The B-vitamins present in oats include B1 (thiamin), B5 (pantothenic acid), folic acid and biotin. These aid metabolism and help regulate energy release from food as well as maintaining a healthy nervous system. Calcium is required to build strong bones and teeth; magnesium is important in the prevention and alleviation of allergies; and iron supports growth and development and aids the production of antibodies and white blood cells, which protect your child from infection.

Like other wholegrains, oats contain the phytonutrient phytic acid. Studies suggest that phytic acid may be able to inhibit the growth of cancer cells and reduce the rate at which they spread. Phytic acid is present in all wholegrains but it does have one down side: it can reduce mineral absorption. For this reason, it is important to eat wholegrains, including oats, within a varied diet.

Oats are also rich in a protein called avenin, which is similar to gluten. Coeliac disease (see pages 132–3) is caused by gluten intolerance and sufferers are advised to avoid oats along with other gluten grains. However, recent studies have shown that they may be able to tolerate avenin as it differs in structure to gluten. It is always wise to check with your doctor if any of your children are coeliacs.

Using oats in your child's diet

As oats are easily digested, they are an excellent grain to introduce to a baby as porridge at around eight months. There are several different oat products used today. *Oat groats* are the whole oat grain, hulled and roasted. These are eaten like rice and take 35–40 minutes to cook. *Steel cut oats* are whole oats that have been chopped up to reduce the cooking time. *Rolled oats*, commonly used in flapjack recipes, are flattened oat kernels that have been steamed to speed up cooking time. *Porridge oats* are oat kernels that have been steamed and flattened even thinner than rolled oats and take even less time to cook. *Oatmeal*, which can also be used to make porridge or oat cakes, comes in different grades; pinhead, rough, medium rough, medium, fine and super-fine. *Oat flour* is ground to a fine powder, thinner than super-fine oatmeal, which is still grainy.

IMMUNE PROFILE

★ B-VITAMINS, VITAMIN E; CALCIUM, IRON, MAGNESIUM, MANGANESE, POTASSIUM, ZINC; FIBRE

▨ PHYTIC ACID

✓ ANTICARCINOGENIC, ANTIOXIDANT

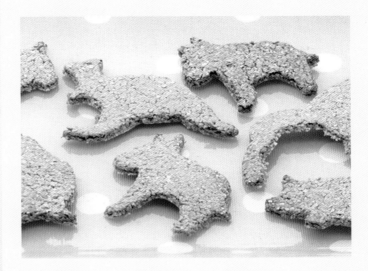

animal oatcakes

makes 15-20 shapes

These are delicious as an accompaniment to soup or as a snack covered in nut butters, or dips such as Quick and Easy Hummus (page 21), Beany Dip (page 21) or Smoked Mackered Dip (page 96).

1 cup (175 g/6 oz) oatmeal
½ tsp bicarbonate of soda
1 tbsp sunflower oil
6–8 tbsp boiling water

Preheat oven to 180°C/350°F/Gas Mark 4. Combine the oatmeal and bicarbonate of soda and sieve them into a mixing bowl. Mix together the oil and water and add to the oatmeal to form a dough. Allow the dough to stand for a few minutes and then roll out on a surface covered with oatmeal. Using pastry cutters or animal shapes cut out shapes and place on a lightly-oiled baking tray. Bake for 25 minutes. Do not allow to brown. Once cooked, allow to cool and then store in a biscuit tin.

oat smoothie

makes 2 large glasses or 4 small

2 bananas
1 cup (350 g/12 oz) soya yoghurt or oatmilk (or natural yoghurt if dairy-tolerant)
1 heaped tbsp rolled oats
1 tbsp honey
1 tbsp linseed (flaxseed) oil
1 cup of ice cubes

Whizz all the ingredients up in a blender and serve immediately.

meat, fish and dairy

CHICKEN

★ B-VITAMINS; IRON, ZINC

✓ ANTIOXIDANT, LOW IN SATURATED FAT

Chicken is one of the most popular meats with children. The darker meat, especially, is high in iron, which supports a healthy immune system and aids your child's general growth and development. Chicken also contains the antioxidant zinc, which helps to protect your child against infection. Recent studies have shown that chicken soup has properties that appear to slow mucus production during illness and can be particularly beneficial for respiratory complaints. Chicken must be cooked thoroughly to prevent possible salmonella poisoning. It is an extremely versatile food and can be stir-fried, roasted, minced, baked, grilled or added to soups and stews.

RECIPES: *chicken and coconut curry (page 64); chicken casserole (page 72); finger lickin' chicken with BBQ sauce (page 88); chicken with butternut squash and coconut (page 96); chicken noodle soup (page 109)*

TURKEY

★ B-VITAMINS; IRON, ZINC

✓ ANTIOXIDANT, LOW IN SATURATED FAT

Turkey is a meat associated with Christmas and Thanksgiving. It is, however, a fantastic food to feed your children throughout the year. Turkey contains more zinc than chicken, and this antioxidant boosts your child's immune system by producing white blood cells and fighting free radicals. This is especially useful during the winter when there are more colds and infections around. Turkey can be roasted, made into burgers or used in stir-fries, soups and stews.

RECIPES: *turkey and cranberry burgers (page 79)*

COD

★ VITAMIN B12; POTASSIUM, SELENIUM

✓ ANTIOXIDANT, LOW IN FAT

Cod is a mild and meaty fish, which is often popular with children. As fish is potentially an allergic food, it is advisable to introduce it to your child with caution, especially if there is a history of food allergies in the family. Cod contains the antioxidant selenium, which helps your child fight infection, and potassium, which boosts energy and is important for heart, muscle and nerve health. Cod can be baked, added to fish pies and stews or made into fishcakes.

RECIPES: *cod and veggies (page 73); toddler fish pie (page 79); cod and parma ham parcels with red pesto (page 89); fish parcels (page 96)*

FRESH ANCHOVY

★ VITAMINS B12 AND D; SELENIUM; OMEGA-3 EFAS

✓ ANTI-ALLERGENIC, ANTI-INFLAMMATORY, ANTIOXIDANT

Anchovies are small fish that are an excellent source of omega-3 essential fatty acids. These EFAs cannot be manufactured by the body, so need to be obtained through diet. They convert into chemicals that regulate the key fighters in your child's immune system, the white blood cells. Today, you can buy fresh anchovies in supermarkets, usually in oil and garlic. These do not have the strong salty taste of the tinned variety and contain far less sodium. As such, they are more palatable to children. Fresh anchovies are particularly delicious added to a salad or combined in a dip.

RECIPES: *anchoiade (page 57); sardine, anchovy and spinach pâté (page 65); hot salad with balsamic dressing and fresh anchovies (page 98)*

FRESH TUNA

★ VITAMINS B3, B12 AND D; SELENIUM; OMEGA-3 EFAS

✓ ANTI-ALLERGENIC, ANTI-INFLAMMATORY, ANTIOXIDANT

Fresh tuna, like other oily fish, is rich in omega-3 essential fatty acids, which play a vital role in protecting the health of your child's immune system. Tinned tuna contains little of these oils but can be a convenient substitute for instant meals. As well as playing an important part in regulating the cells of the immune system, omega-3 essential fats are naturally anti-inflammatory and can be used therapeutically in allergic conditions such as eczema, and in autoimmune conditions such as ulcerative colitis and rheumatoid arthritis. Owing to the current pollution levels in the seas, tuna and other oily fish should not be given to a child more than once a week. Fresh tuna can be grilled, made into fish cakes or combined with vegetables and pasta or rice.

RECIPES: *tuna fishcakes (page 79); make your own pizza (page 80); tuna and prawn brochette with coriander marinade (page 89)*

MACKEREL

★ B-VITAMINS, VITAMIN D; SELENIUM; OMEGA-3 EFAS

✓ ANTI-ALLERGENIC, ANTI-INFLAMMATORY, ANTIOXIDANT

Mackerel is an oily fish that is another excellent source of omega-3 essential fatty acids. These EFAs help to regulate the activity of the immune army and have anti-inflammatory properties. Mackerel is also a good source of selenium, an antioxidant that helps protect your child from infection and free-radical damage. Selenium is also anticarcinogenic and is found in all seafood. Mackerel has a strong taste and is therefore best combined with other fish or flavours.

RECIPES: smoked mackerel dip (page 96)

PRAWN

★ VITAMIN B12; SELENIUM

✓ ANTICARCINOGENIC, ANTIOXIDANT

Prawns are a type of shellfish. They contain good levels of the antioxidant selenium, often lacking in our diets, which helps to protect the immune system from free-radical damage and also has anticarcinogenic properties. Prawns or, indeed, any shellfish should not be introduced to your child before the age of two as they can trigger allergic reactions in susceptible people. If there is a family history of shellfish allergy, it is wise to avoid it altogether. Prawns can be grilled, added to fish pies, soups and stews or used in stir-fries.

RECIPES: quick and easy seafood pasta supper (page 63); tuna and prawn brochette with coriander marinade (page 89); sweet and sour prawn stir-fry with egg noodles and bok choi (page 96); family paella (page 98)

SQUID

★ B-VITAMINS, VITAMIN E; SELENIUM

✓ ANTICARCINOGENIC, ANTIOXIDANT

Squid, like octopus, is part of the cephalopod family and is an excellent source of the antioxidant selenium. Together with the antioxidant vitamin E, selenium helps to protect the immune system from free-radical damage. Vitamin E also helps to maintain healthy cell membranes in your child's body. Squid has a meaty, chewy texture that can be popular with children. It can be grilled whole or sliced and added to stir-fries or paellas.

RECIPES: seafood paella (page 66)

EGG

★ VITAMINS A, B12 AND D; IRON

✓ ANTI-ANAEMIC, ANTIOXIDANT

Eggs are a rich source of vitamin A, which helps to protect your child from respiratory and other infections. Vitamin A is also required for the proper production of fighter cells in your child's immune army. Eggs are also high in iron, which boosts energy and immunity. However, the iron in eggs is not easily aborbed by your child's body, so eggs should be served with a vitamin C-rich food, such as a glass of orange juice, as vitamin C aids iron absorption. Eggs can be scrambled, boiled, poached, or used in baking.

RECIPES: smoked salmon scramble (page 65); parsley eggs (page 78); toddler fish pie (page 79); sweetcorn patties (page 81); muesli squares (page 83); dry-fried eggy bread (page 86); egg and veggie bake (page 90)

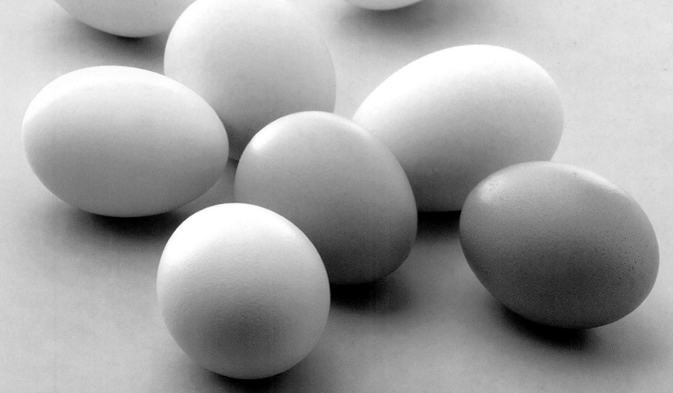

game

GAME IS A WONDERFUL SOURCE OF IMMUNE-BOOSTING NUTRIENTS AND
COMES WITH THE ADDED ADVANTAGE OF BEING FREE FROM THE
ANTIBIOTICS AND HORMONES GIVEN TO MOST FARMED ANIMALS.

Origins

The hunting of game (wild animals) has been documented from the
time of the first appearance of humans 100,000 years ago. Then,
all animals were wild and hunting was a major part of life. For the
purposes of this book, game describes venison, duck, pheasant,
partridge, grouse, quail, guinea fowl and wood pigeon. Wild game
is free from the antibiotics, hormones and growth promoters
routinely administered to farmed animals. Owing to the nature of
its environment, game is also extremely lean as it has freedom to
roam and does not build up fat reserves like farmed animals.
However, some game, such as duck and venison, is increasingly
available in farmed varieties, so it is advisable to check your source
of game to make sure it is wild
wherever possible.

Immune-boosting profile

Game provides plenty of protein and B-vitamins in your child's diet.
Protein contains all the amino acids needed to repair tissue and
build new cells. Eating too much animal protein has been associated
with a higher risk of degenerative diseases, but, taking into account
all of its other nutritional benefits, including game that is in season
in your child's diet once or twice a week is a good balance.

The B-group of vitamins are vital for the process of metabolism
– converting food into energy. Each B-vitamin has an important role
to play in your child's health. Vitamin B1 is essential for energy
production, digestion and proper brain function. Vitamin B2 is
important for turning protein, fat and sugars into energy. It is also
needed for healthy eyes, skin and hair. Vitamin B3 helps metabolize
carbohydrates and keeps the digestive and nervous systems
operating well. It also plays a key role in balancing blood sugar
levels. Vitamin B5 is an important "stress" vitamin. It is involved in
producing anti-stress hormones, as well as being a co-factor in
energy production. Vitamin B6 is required for protein metabolism

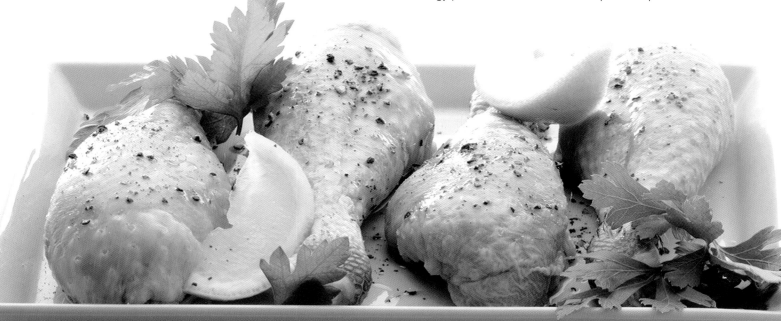

and for the production and balance of sex hormones. It is also involved in fatty acid metabolism and helps in the control of allergic reactions. Vitamin B12 is needed for energy production and a healthy nervous system. Biotin is a B vitamin important for healthy skin and hair, as well as assisting in essential fatty acid metabolism. Folic acid, another member of the B-group, is vital during pregnancy for the development of the brain and nerves of the unborn child. It is also involved in protein metabolism and red blood cell production. Skin and hair problems, lack of energy and nervous disorders can all be symptoms of B-vitamin deficiency.

Game is also an excellent source of iron, a particularly important mineral for growing children. Venison, for example, contains three times as much iron as lamb, and pheasant has almost four times the amount found in beef. Iron is needed for the production of white blood cells, a key part of your child's immune army. Iron deficiency (anaemia) is quite common among toddlers and teenagers owing to poor diet, causing slow development and susceptibility to infection.

Game is rich in the antioxidant zinc, another immune booster that helps protect your child from free-radical damage as well as preventing infection. Zinc is required for healthy metabolism and growth and for the proper formation of the nervous system in unborn babies. Zinc deficiency in children can be detected by looking at their fingernails. If they have more than three white spots on their nails, you can suspect a zinc deficiency. Other symptoms are reduced appetite and a poor sense of taste and smell.

Using game in your child's diet

Game should be eaten fresh rather than frozen wherever possible. Avoid the farmed varieties unless you are confident of your source, as they may have been subjected to the same intensive farming practices as other livestock.

Game can be roasted, braised or casseroled. Pheasant is mild tasting, rather like chicken and is a cheap form of poultry when in season. Venison makes a deliciously rich casserole served with lashings of mashed potato and green beans. Venison can now be bought in sausage form, as mince, as a joint or as casserole meat. Duck is another popular variety of game. It can be roasted or stir-fried in strips served with noodles and stir-fried vegetables.

IMMUNE PROFILE

★ B-VITAMINS; IRON, ZINC

✓ ANTI-ANAEMIC, ANTIOXIDANT

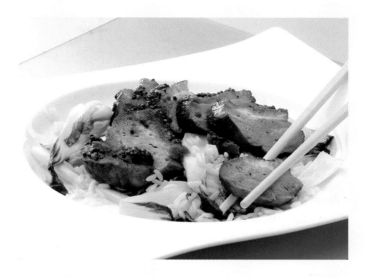

glazed duck with honey and mustard

2 tbsp wholegrain mustard
2 tbsp runny honey
4 duck breasts, skinned

Preheat the oven 190°C/375°F/Gas Mark 5. In a dish, mix the mustard and honey marinade and coat the duck with it. Place the duck in a lightly-oiled roasting pan and pour over any remaining marinade. Cover and bake for 20 minutes or until cooked through. Leave the duck to sit for a few minutes before serving over some rice and stir-fried bok choi.

braised broth of guinea fowl with winter vegetables

1 guinea fowl
1 tbsp extra virgin olive oil
1 onion, chopped
1 packet of chopped pancetta
2 leeks, chopped
2 garlic cloves, crushed
A couple of sage leaves
A couple of sprigs of thyme
850 ml (1½ pints) vegetable stock
A handful of pearl barley
12 baby carrots
2 medium potatoes, sliced
A handful of chopped flat leaf parsley

Preheat oven to 180°C/350°F/Gas Mark 4. In a heavy casserole pan, heat the oil and lightly brown the guinea fowl (which looks like a small chicken). Remove the guinea fowl and add the onion, pancetta, leeks, garlic, sage and thyme and cook them for a few minutes until they have softened. Return the guinea fowl and cover with the vegetable stock. Add the pearl barley and carrots and place the sliced potatoes over the guinea fowl. Cover and bake in the oven for 1 hour. Remove lid and cook for another 30 minutes to brown the guinea fowl and any potatoes on top. Once cooked, the meat should fall off the bones with ease. Spoon off any excess fat, break up the guinea fowl and remove the bones. Sprinkle with chopped flat leaf parsley and serve in soup bowls.

salmon

FRESH SALMON IS RICH IN ANTIOXIDANT VITAMINS AND MINERALS AS WELL AS OMEGA-3 ESSENTIAL FATTY ACIDS, ALL OF WHICH PLAY AN IMPORTANT ROLE IN THE HEALTH OF YOUR CHILD'S IMMUNE SYSTEM.

Origins

Salmon belong to the *Salmonidae* family of fish and, in the wild, their natural habitats are the Atlantic and Pacific oceans. These are home to several types of salmon. The Atlantic salmon is called the *Salmo salar* and Pacific varieties include the Chinook, sockeye, pink, coho and chum. The lifestyle of the salmon is remarkable and as yet not fully understood. They are anadromous fish, which means that they leave their saltwater homes to lay their eggs in freshwater rivers. They begin their lives as eggs on the gravely bottom of a cold stream. As the fish grow, they adapt to be able to live in sea water as well as freshwater and make their journey down towards the sea. They spend on average two to four years at sea before finding their way back upstream on a long and arduous journey to lay their eggs. It is during this return journey that fishermen normally catch the salmon.

In the late 20th century, fish farming, especially of salmon, became popular. It increased the availability of fish to eat but led to a sharp decline in its quality as mass-farming practices, such as overcrowding and overuse of routine pesticides and antibiotics, became widespread. In the last few years, as many as one in ten farmed salmon has been found to contain raised levels of pesticides that can be toxic and potentially harmful to human health. For this reason it is always better to buy wild or organic farmed salmon in order to maximize the benefits received from eating this tasty fish.

Immune-boosting profile

Salmon is rich in the vitamins A, B12 and D, as well as the mineral selenium. Vitamin A is an antioxidant, which means it neutralizes harmful free radical atoms that can cause disease in your child's body. It also plays a vital role in protecting the body's mucous membranes and in essential fatty acid metabolism. Vitamin A is found only in animal sources but the body is able to make it from beta-carotene food sources if it is otherwise unavailable. Vitamin B12 is one of the B-group of water-soluble vitamins. It helps to keep the blood and nervous systems healthy and supports normal growth and development. Vitamin D aids calcium absorption and is good for general bone health. Selenium is another powerful antioxidant that also helps to produce antibodies.

Salmon is an excellent source of omega-3 essential fatty acids (EFAs), and it is for this reason that it gets most of its good publicity. Salmon is often discussed together with other oily fish, such as tuna, mackerel and herring, because they are all rich sources of omega-3 EFAs. Along with omega-6 group EFAs (found in sunflower, safflower, evening primrose and corn oils), these fatty acids play a very important role in the health of your children. They are called essential because the body cannot manufacture them; they have to be acquired through diet.

In the presence of certain vitamins and minerals, including vitamin A and selenium, EFAs convert into hormone-like chemical messengers called prostaglandins, which play an important role in immune health. They regulate the activity of the white blood cells of the immune army and exhibit anti-inflammatory properties, useful in combating such conditions as eczema and arthritis. In addition, omega-3 fats, which can also be found in linseed oil, walnut and walnut oil, and soyabean and wheatgerm oils, specifically convert into prostaglandins that are essential for proper brain development and function. A lack of these oils has been implicated as a contributing factor in common childhood conditions such as hyperactivity, learning difficulties, dyslexia and dyspraxia. Omega-3 essential fatty acids also serve to protect your child from disease in later life. They help to control cholesterol and fat levels, thereby protecting the cardiovascular system and reducing the risk of heart disease and other circulatory problems.

Using salmon in your child's diet

There has recently been a great deal of publicity regarding pollution problems in the sea and the consequent fish contamination. In addition, farmed salmon has had its share of bad press, too. Try to buy salmon from a reliable, non-farmed source wherever possible. Generally, the best defence in this ever increasing chemical age is to arm your children with a strong immune system and feed them a diet rich in nutrients that can deal with any chemical residues they inevitably encounter daily. Reliably-sourced oily fish, like salmon, can help this battle if included in your child's diet once a week.

Salmon is a popular fish with children. It is safe to introduce to your baby from six months. However, if your family has any history of food allergies, especially to fish, it would be wise to wait until your child is over a year old. Mixed with other fish, salmon is one of the milder tasting oily fish. It can be made into fish cakes, lightly steamed and served with vegetables, or added to stir-fries and other fish dishes such as fish pie.

IMMUNE PROFILE

★ VITAMINS A, B12 AND D; SELENIUM; OMEGA-3 FATS

✓ ANTI-ALLERGENIC, ANTICARCINOGENIC, ANTI-INFLAMMATORY,

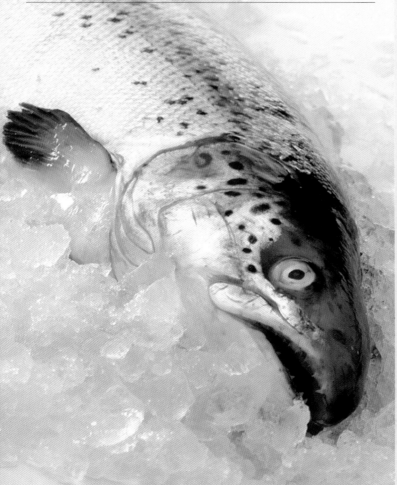

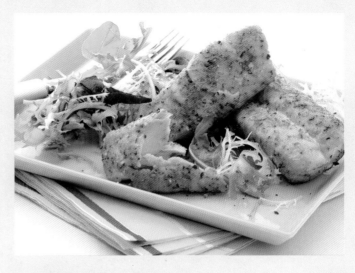

fresh salmon fish cakes

makes 8 small fish cakes

These make a pleasant change from cod.

2 small salmon fillets, skinless and boneless
4 small potatoes, peeled and chopped
1 medium onion, finely chopped
2 tbsp extra virgin olive oil
1 egg, beaten
A small handful of parsley, chopped

Bake or steam the salmon for 20 minutes until cooked through. Meanwhile, boil and lightly mash the potatoes. Sauté the onion in about half of the olive oil until soft. Mix all the ingredients together and form into eight small fishcakes. Place in the fridge for 1 hour before cooking. Gently fry in the rest of the olive oil until crisp on both sides.

salmon fish fingers

makes 12 fish fingers

1 tsp dried mixed herbs
A large handful of ground almonds or sesame seeds
2 chunky salmon fillets, skinless and boneless, cut into thick fingers
2 tbsp extra virgin olive oil

Combine the mixed herbs together with the ground almonds in a shallow dish. Roll the salmon fingers in the mixture until they are coated. In a frying pan, gently cook the fish in the olive oil for 5–10 minutes, depending on the thickness of the salmon fillet. Keep turning the fish fingers to ensure they are evenly cooked right through.

yoghurt

YOGHURT IS A LIVING FOOD THAT PROVIDES EASILY ABSORBED NUTRIENTS AND BENEFICIAL BACTERIA VITAL FOR YOUR CHILD'S INTESTINAL HEALTH AND IMMUNE SYSTEM.

Origins

Yoghurt was probably first discovered, by accident, by nomadic Balkan tribes 4,000 years ago. It is created from milk through a fermentation process facilitated by friendly bacteria on lactose (milk sugars). The most common strains of bacteria used in this process are *Lactobacillus bulgaricus* and *Streptoccocus thermophilus*. The lactose is converted into lactic acid, which thickens the milk and creates yoghurt's slightly sour, tangy taste. Yoghurt supplies the same nutrients as milk but the live cultures it contains make it easier to digest, resulting in better absorption levels of these nutrients in the body. Yoghurt can also be made from non-dairy products such as soya milk and this would carry the same excellent health benefits as milk yoghurt.

Today, there is a plethora of yoghurt products available to buy and this can cause some confusion. A few definitions are helpful. All yoghurt will contain some live bacteria unless it has been pasteurized or heat-treated after it has been made. "Bio-yoghurts" are those to which extra bacteria have been added to further enhance their nutritional benefit. However, some commercial varieties of live yoghurts and bio-yoghurts have been tested and found to contain friendly bacteria that are more dead than alive. So, in order to reap the benefits of the live bacteria, it is probably safer to make your own yoghurt (see right). Fruit yoghurts, whether claiming to contain live bacteria or not, are usually laden with sugar, an immuno-suppressant. Some popular brands available in supermarkets have as much as four teaspoons of sugar in one small pot. "Natural" yoghurt and "plain" yoghurt mean the same thing, simply that they are not a fruit variety. Basically, in terms of your child's health, you cannot beat plain, live, natural yoghurt to which you can add fruit, fruit purée or honey.

Immune-boosting profile

Yoghurt contains *lactobacillus* bacteria, which are hugely beneficial to your child's bowel health. We all have bacteria in our small and large intestines. Some are good, beneficial bacteria and some are rogue bacteria that can do us harm if they become more prevalent than the good (as in the case of *Candida Albicans* see page 104). The ratios of these bacteria differ for each of us depending on whether we were breastfed or bottle fed, our age, which diseases and bugs we have been exposed to and whether or not we have taken any antibiotics. The good bacteria, *lactobacillus* and

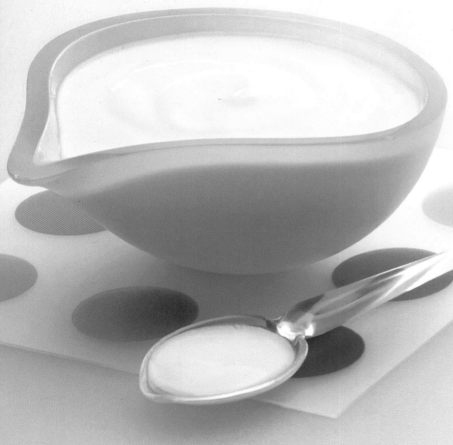

bifidobacteria, are part of your child's first line of defence against harmful bacteria and viruses. They are often referred to as probiotics. They are also important as they produce certain B-vitamins, aid digestion, protect against tummy bugs and food poisoning, and improve overall resistance to disease. These bacteria also make substances called bacteriocins, which act as natural antibiotics and kill off undesirable microbes (disease-causing bacteria). Antibiotics can wipe out these beneficial bacteria for up to six months but yoghurt helps to replenish the body's supply, so giving it to your child regularly after a course of antibiotics is a great way of redressing the balance.

Yoghurt is also full of calcium, which is required for strong bones and teeth. An added bonus is that the calcium contained in yoghurt is far more easily absorbed than that found in other forms of dairy produce. Calcium is also an important mineral for proper immune function. It is needed by the complement system, which is a collection of proteins that can destroy unwanted bacteria.

Using yoghurt in your child's diet

Owing to its easy digestibility, yoghurt is an excellent first dairy product to introduce to your child. Mixed with fruit purée, it makes a delicious pudding without the sugar, colours and thickening agents added to commercial yoghurts. It is quick and easy to make at home and this is an activity that older children will enjoy helping you with. Yoghurt can also be used to replace cream for a healthier accompaniment to puddings, and can be added to smoothies to give creaminess to the texture and boost nutritional content. Yoghurt is not ideal for high-heat cooking as it curdles easily but it can be used as a very effective meat tenderizer, owing to its lactic acid, as in the case of Indian dishes like tandoori chicken.

Many people who are intolerant to dairy products find that they are able to eat yoghurt. For those who can't, you can make soya yoghurt or buy it at most supermarkets. If a child is allergic to dairy and soya products, you can now buy probiotics in powdered form, which can be added to smoothies and juices. This is a useful form of the beneficial bacteria needed to replenish that lost should your child have to take antibiotics. As these products contain live bacteria, they should be bought refrigerated and kept in the fridge.

IMMUNE PROFILE

★ VITAMINS B2 AND B12; CALCIUM, POTASSIUM

✓ AIDS DIGESTION, ANTIBACTERIAL

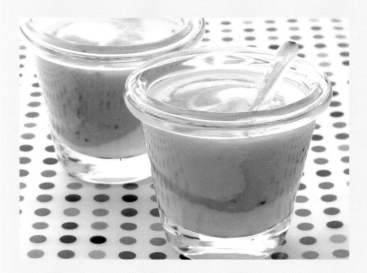

homemade yoghurt with four fruit purée

600 ml (1 pint) whole milk
1 tbsp live yoghurt
4 tbsp skimmed milk powder
1 mango, peeled and destoned
2 bananas, peeled
1 papaya, peeled and deseeded
1 kiwi fruit, peeled

Put a couple of tablespoons of the milk into a measuring jug. Add the yoghurt and mix well. In a saucepan, whisk the skimmed milk powder into the remaining milk. Heat to boiling point, then remove from the heat and allow to cool until you can put your finger into it. Pour the milk over the yoghurt, stirring all the time. Pour into a bowl, cover with a clean tea towel and leave in a warm place overnight until set. Once set, keep in the fridge and use within a week. For the four fruit purée, whizz up all of the fruit in a blender until smooth. To make up the pudding, simply put a spoonful of yoghurt in a bowl and add a spoonful of purée on top.

homemade soya yoghurt

600 ml (1 pint) of soya milk
1 tbsp live soya yoghurt

Put two tablespoons of the milk in a jug and add the soya yoghurt. Heat the remaining milk in a saucepan and bring to the boil. Remove from the heat and leave to cool. Pour the milk over the yoghurt, stirring all the time. Pour into a bowl, cover with a clean tea towel and leave in a warm place overnight until set. Once set, keep in the fridge and use within a week.

almond lassi

makes 2 large glasses or 4 small ones

Lassi is a deliciously light yoghurt drink that originated in India.

1 cup (225 ml/8 fl oz) live yoghurt
½ tsp natural almond essence
⅓ cup (40 g/1½ oz) flaked almonds
1 cup of ice cubes
1–2 tbsp honey

Whizz all the ingredients up together in a blender and serve straightaway.

pulses and beans

BUTTER BEAN

★ IRON, ZINC; FIBRE

✓ CHOLESTEROL LOWERING

Butter beans are mild tasting and a good source of vegetable protein. They contain useful amounts of iron and zinc, which your child's immune system needs to operate efficiently. Butter beans also contain plenty of soluble fibre. This helps to remove cholesterol from the gut and prevent constipation. Butter beans can be bought dried, in which case they need to be soaked overnight to rehydrate them, and then cooked for 90 minutes. Alternatively, they can be bought in a tin, but try to get the no added salt or sugar varieties. Butter beans are delicious added to soups or stews.

RECIPES: coconut and cauliflower soup (page 63)

CHICKPEA

★ FOLIC ACID, VITAMIN E; IRON, MANGANESE

▨ ISOFLAVONES, SAPONINS

✓ ANTICARCINOGENIC, ANTIOXIDANT, CHOLESTEROL LOWERING

Chickpeas contain phytonutrients called saponins, which are antioxidants that have anti-cancer effects. They work by stimulating the immune system and blocking the development of cancer cells. Saponins also lower cholesterol. Chickpeas are a good vegetarian source of protein and are the main ingredient in hummus. They can be bought dried or tinned. The dried variety must be soaked overnight and cooked for 90 minutes. Alternatively, you can buy the tinned variety that have no added salt or sugar. Chickpeas can be added to soups, salads or casseroles.

RECIPES: quick and easy hummus (page 21); handy hummus with baked potato (page 74); rustic saturday soup (page 95)

GREEN AND BROWN LENTILS

★ FOLIC ACID; IRON, SELENIUM, ZINC; FIBRE

▨ ISOFLAVONES, LIGNANS

✓ ANTICARCINOGENIC, ANTIOXIDANT

Green lentils are a rich vegetable source of iron. This is needed for the production of white blood cells, the lynchpins of your child's immune system. Lentils are also an ideal food during pregnancy because of their high levels of iron and folic acid, important for energy and healthy foetal development. Lentils are also rich in the antioxidants zinc and selenium, which protect your child from free-radical damage. Green and brown lentils make good alternatives to meat in dishes such as shepherd's pie and burgers.

RECIPES: farmhouse lentil pie (page 82); the very best vegetarian burgers (page 86)

RED LENTIL

★ BETA-CAROTENE, FOLIC ACID; IRON, ZINC; FIBRE

▨ ISOFLAVONES, LIGNANS, PHYTATES

✓ ANTICARCINOGENIC, ANTIOXIDANT

All lentils are a rich source of iron for vegetarians. In addition, red lentils also contain beta-carotene, a potent antioxidant and the vegetable form of vitamin A, which helps to strengthen your child's immune defences. The fibre in lentils maintains a healthy bowel, and the phytonutrients they contain have anti-cancer properties. Red lentils are very quick and easy to cook. They make an excellent purée for babies and are delicious added to soups and stews for older children.

RECIPES: hearty lentil soup (page 62); warming lentil and potato bake (page 64); immune-boosting lentil purée (page 73)

SOYA BEAN

★ VITAMIN E; CALCIUM, IRON, MAGNESIUM, ZINC

▨ ISOFLAVONES

✓ ANTICARCINOGENIC, ANTIOXIDANT, BONE STRENGTHING

Soya beans are the most nutritious of all beans and contain more protein weight for weight than any other food of vegetable or animal origin. They contain calcium, so are good for bones and teeth, and are packed with anticarcinogenic antioxidants. Soya comes in many forms: soya beans, soya flour, soya milk, tofu, tempeh, soy sauce and miso, soya yoghurt, soya cheese and soya cream. Delicious in oriental cooking, soya products are also a useful dairy alternative.

RECIPES: homemade soya yoghurt (page 51); protein shake (page 62); smoked salmon scramble (page 65); tempting tofu pasta sauce (page 74); protein shake (page 129); oatbran and berries smoothie (page 131)

herbs, spices and condiments

CHILLI

★ BETA-CAROTENE, VITAMIN C

▨ CAPSAICIN

✓ ANTI-INFLAMMATORY, ANTIOXIDANT, ANTISEPTIC, DECONGESTANT

Over the centuries, chillies have been used therapeutically both to help prevent and to treat disease. All chillies contain capsaicin, a phytonutrient with both antioxidant and anti-inflammatory properties. Like ginger, cloves, horseradish, garlic and mustard, chilli has an antiseptic and expectorant action on the respiratory system, helping to shift mucus, making it an excellent decongestant for colds, cataarh and sinus problems. Chillies and chilli powder should be added only in tiny amounts when feeding young children owing to its intense heat. Older children may enjoy hot food and, therefore, derive a greater benefit from chillies' medicinal properties.

RECIPES: *rustic saturday soup (page 95); magnesium broth (page 103); immune-boosting chicken broth (page 126)*

CINNAMON

★ CALCIUM, IRON, MAGNESIUM,

▨ EUGENOL

✓ ANALGESIC, ANTISEPTIC, DECONGESTANT

Research suggests that cinnamon has the ability to inhibit viruses. It also acts as a nasal decongestant and these properties, together with its warming quality, make cinnamon a useful spice in the treatment of colds and flu. In addition, cinnamon contains the phytonutrient eugenol, which has both antiseptic and analgesic properties. Cinnamon is a delicious ingredient in many sweet and savoury dishes, and a stick of cinnamon is a great addition to a hot toddy that may help ward off a cold.

RECIPES: *venison steaks with baked butternut squash and cinnamon (page 63); chicken and coconut curry (page 64); baked apple with raisins and spices (page 75); banana and raisin cake (page 83); healthy apple strudel (page 99)*

CLOVE

★ VITAMIN C

▨ EUGENOL

✓ ANALGESIC, ANTIOXIDANT, ANTISEPTIC, ANTIVIRAL

Cloves have powerful antiseptic qualities capable of inhibiting viruses and fungi. Like cinnamon, they contain a substance called eugenol, which not only gives their distinctive aroma but also provides their analgesic and antiseptic properties. Clove oil has for centuries been used as a treatment for tooth and gum infections. Cloves are an effective expectorant and this, combined with their warming action and antioxidant vitamin C, can offer a useful treatment for colds and coughs. Cloves make an excellent addition to puddings such as fruit crumbles, rice puddings or stewed apple.

RECIPES: *chicken and coconut curry (page 64); stewed apple purée with cloves and molasses (page 72); clove tea (page 107)*

CORIANDER

★ BETA-CAROTENE, FOLIC ACID; IRON

▨ CHLOROPHYLL, CORIANDROL

✓ ANTICARCINOGENIC, ANTIOXIDANT

Also known as "chinese parsley", coriander leaves and seeds have traditionally been used to treat urinary complaints and as a tonic for the digestive system. Coriander is very popular in Middle Eastern and Asian food and is a good source of chlorophyll, the phytonutrient in all green vegetables that is believed to protect against cancer. Coriander contains coriandrol, a phytonutrient that early research indicates can combat liver cancer. Fresh coriander is delicious chopped and sprinkled on soups, salads and casseroles. Ground coriander is a main ingredient in curry powder.

RECIPES: *hearty lentil soup (page 62); chicken and coconut curry (page 64); roasted vegetables with coriander couscous (page 65); immune-boosting lentil purée (page 73); sweetcorn patties (page 81); tuna and prawn brochette with coriander marinade (page 89); fish parcels (page 96)*

FRUCTOSE (FRUIT SUGAR)

Although fructose contains no really useful nutrients for your child, it is a helpful alternative to refined white sugar. It looks and tastes like ordinary sugar but, although it is easily digested, it is described as a slow-releasing sugar. This is because your child's body cannot utilize fructose as it is. It can only use glucose and, in order to use the fructose sugar, it has to convert it into this form. This takes time, thereby slowing down the release of sugar into your child's bloodstream and avoiding the sugar highs and lows that can result from eating too much refined sugar. Also, fructose is extremely sweet and can be used in smaller amounts than refined white sugar. Like any sugar, fructose should be used sparingly to prevent dental caries and its immune-suppressive effects.

RECIPES: *ginger cake (page 66); blackcurrant ice cream (page 90); homemade digestive biscuits (page 91); fresh lemonade (page 119); gluten-free chocolate brownie birthday cake (page 133)*

GINGER

★ B-VITAMINS; MAGNESIUM, ZINC

✓ ANTIOXIDANT, ANTISEPTIC, DECONGESTANT

Ginger is a warming antiseptic spice. Strong, fresh ginger tea, made simply by infusing a piece of ginger root in a mug of hot water, can help stop a cold in its tracks. Ginger is also an expectorant and a decongestant. As such, it helps to break down mucus and provides relief for conditions such as sinusitis and bronchitis. Ginger tastes great added to stir-fries and oriental dishes. It also blends well with sweet foods and can be added to puddings and smoothies.

RECIPES: *warming lentil and potato bake (page 64); chicken and coconut curry (page 64); ginger cake (page 66); stir-fry duck strips with orange and ginger (page 97); queen scallop stir-fry (page 98); watermelon and ginger ice (page 98); ginger and pear crumble (page 99); ginger toddy (page 103)*

MANUKA HONEY

✓ ANTIBACTERIAL, ANTISEPTIC, ANTIVIRAL

Manuka, or tea tree, honey, is a must for every family's kitchen cupboard because of its incredible antibacterial and antiviral properties. This honey helps to soothe sore throats and can even be applied to cuts and grazes. It is now used medicinally in Australian hospitals to treat wounds. Do not give honey to children under the age of one year as there is a small risk of infection.

RECIPES: *ginger toddy (page 103); thyme and honey tea (page 107); clove tea (page 107); almond milk (page 113); garlic and honey syrup (page 125)*

MINT

★ BETA-CAROTENE, FOLIC ACID, VITAMINS C AND E

▨ CHOROPHYLL, LIMONENE

✓ ANTIBACTERIAL, ANTICARCINOGENIC, ANTIOXIDANT, ANTIVIRAL

There are many different varieties of mint and each has its own aroma and flavour. Mint has antiviral and antibacterial properties and is a useful herb to take when there are colds and flu around. Mint is calming to the digestive system and peppermint tea can help to relieve stomach pains and colic. Mint is also reported to have anti-cancer properties due to the presence of the phytonutrient limonene. An extremely versatile herb, mint is delicious in sweet and savoury foods alike and most children will enjoy its flavour.

RECIPES: *mint and mango smoothie (page 66); venison sausages with pea, mint and potato mash (page 88)*

MOLASSES

★ CALCIUM, IRON, POTASSIUM

Molasses is a by-product of the sugar-refining process and is well known for its high level of minerals. Weight for weight, molasses contains more calcium than milk and more iron than eggs. It is a good natural sweetener, but has a very strong taste so should be used in small amounts. Children will enjoy molasses drizzled on ice cream, porridge, or blended in a smoothie.

RECIPES: *protein shake (page 62); ginger cake (page 66); stewed apple purée with cloves and molasses (page 72); baked apple with raisins and spices (page 75); creamy cashew porridge (page 78); finger lickin' chicken with BBQ sauce (page 88)*

PARSLEY

★ BETA-CAROTENE, FOLIC ACID, VITAMIN C; IRON, MAGNESIUM

▨ CHLOROPHYLL, COUMARINS

✓ ANTICARCINOGENIC, ANTIOXIDANT

Parsley is the king of herbs! Packed with a heady mix of minerals and antioxidant vitamins and phytonutrients, parsley boosts your child's immune system and wards off infection. Parsley also contains coumarins, phytonutrients that have been found to protect the heart and to inhibit the development of cancer cells, and chlorophyll, which is another anticarcinogen. Parsley can be added to soups and stews, spinkled on salads or even added to homemade juices. Always add parsley at the end of cooking to preserve its colour and nutrients.

RECIPES: venison and shiitake casserole (page 25); smoked salmon scramble (page 65); sardine, anchovy and spinach paté (page 65); immune-boosting lentil purée (page 73); parsley eggs (page 78); toddler fish pie (page 79); farmhouse lentil pie (page 82); smoked mackerel dip (page 96); salmon kedgeree (page 113); immunity soup (page 123)

ROSEMARY

★ BETA-CAROTENE; CALCIUM, POTASSIUM, ZINC

▨ QUINONES, ROSMARINIC ACID

✓ ANTICARCINOGENIC, ANTIOXIDANT, ANTISEPTIC

Rosemary, a Mediterranean herb, contains around 12 free-radical destroying compounds, which activate detoxification enzymes that assist in ridding the body of harmful substances. It has traditionally been used to treat headaches and also as an antiseptic gargle. Rosemary also contains the antioxidants zinc and beta-carotene, as well as quinones, which are phytonutrients that have been shown to inhibit the development of cancer cells. It is delicious with meat or added to roasted vegetables and potatoes.

THYME

★ BETA-CAROTENE; CALCIUM

▨ THYMOL

✓ ANTIBACTERIAL, ANTIOXIDANT, ANTISEPTIC, ANTIVIRAL

Thyme has excellent antibacterial and antiviral properties, which makes it very useful for warding off colds and coughs in the winter months. It also contains an oil, thymol, that has antiseptic qualities. Some studies have shown that thyme can also protect against food poisoning. Thyme is a delicious addition to Mediterranean dishes.

RECIPES: braised broth of guinea fowl with winter vegetables (page 47); venison burgers (page 88); thyme and honey tea (page 107); thyme and chicken casserole (page 107); immunity soup (page 123)

TURMERIC

★ IRON, POTASSIUM

▨ CURCUMIN

✓ ANTICARCINOGENIC, ANTI-INFLAMMATORY

Bright yellow turmeric is a member of the ginger family. It is used primarily in Indian cooking in its dried, powdered form. Turmeric contains the phytonutrient curcumin, which studies have shown to have anti-cancer effects, especially against stomach and colon cancers. Curcumin is also well-documented for its anti-inflammatory properties. Early research has indicated that high doses of

curcumin may be able to slow the development of AIDS by blocking a key protein that is secreted by HIV-infected cells. Turmeric can be added to paella dishes to give colour or mixed with other spices to create a curry powder.

RECIPES: coconut and cauliflower soup (page 63); chicken and coconut curry (page 64); seafood paella (page 66); family paella (page 98)

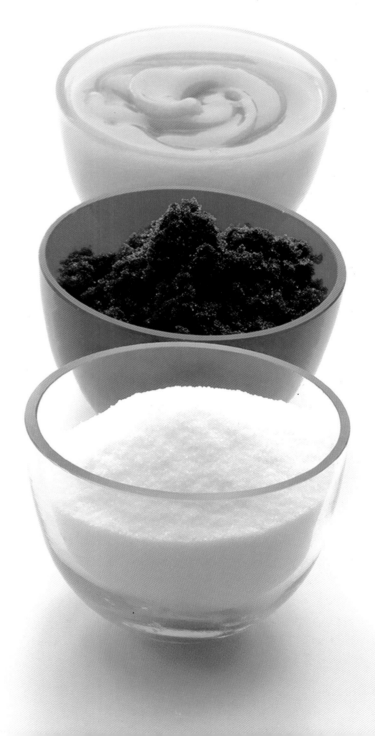

garlic

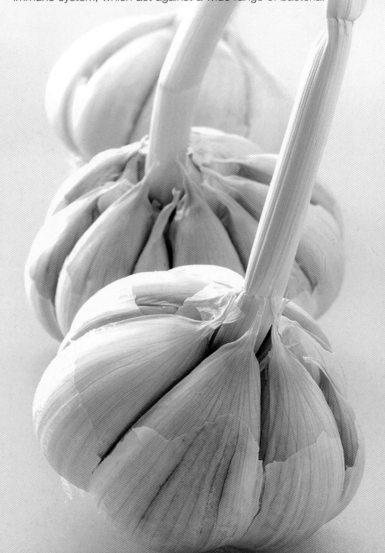

GARLIC IS A SUPERFOOD FOR YOUR CHILD'S IMMUNE SYSTEM. RICH IN SULPHUR COMPOUNDS IT KEEPS BLOOD HEALTHY, HELPS COMBAT BACTERIAL AND FUNGAL INFECTION AND WARDS OFF VIRUSES.

Origins

Garlic (*Allium sativum*) is part of the allium family. Other members include onion, chive, spring onion, shallot and leek. Garlic originates from Central Asia, where it has been cultivated for some 5,000 years. Around 4,500 years ago, in ancient Egypt, garlic was given daily to the pyramid builders, to keep up their strength and ward off contagious diseases. The Ancient Greeks also believed that garlic was a useful defence against illness and old age. It is recorded that in around 776BCE, competitors in the Olympic Games ate garlic regularly to improve performance and stamina. There are many species of wild garlic and it is believed that the cultivated variety we know today may have evolved from species in Asia and the eastern Mediterranean region.

Immune-boosting profile

Garlic's attributes have been well-documented internationally. Louis Pasteur first discovered its antibacterial ability in the 19th century, but it was not until the 1940s that garlic's specific medicinal qualities were isolated. It was then discovered that one of the sulphur compounds present in garlic converted to a powerful phytonutrient, allicin, under enzymatic processes. Allicin is the strong-smelling component of garlic and has been found to be effective at preventing some cancers, such as stomach cancer. It is believed that allicin can inhibit the growth of certain bacteria that are implicated as a major cause of stomach cancer.

Other members of the allium family contain similar sulphur compounds to garlic, which are similarly responsible for their pungent aromas, but none have them in as concentrated a form as garlic. It is for this reason that garlic ranks the highest of all alliums as a superfood for the immune system. Today, garlic is recognized as having clear antibacterial, antiviral and antifungal properties. It has been found to be more effective than 13 other spices against specific bacteria, such as E. coli, which cause food poisoning and urinary infections, and several other lesser-known bacteria. Garlic is truly one of nature's best anti-microbials. This means that it fights disease-causing organisms and it does this by stimulating the production of white blood cells, the vanguard of your child's immune system, which act against a wide range of bacteria.

Garlic has traditionally been used as a medicinal food for treating parasites in the stomach and intestines. Studies have shown that the use of garlic extract proved highly effective in the treatment of children affected by the parasite Giardia and by tapeworm. Other studies have shown garlic to be particularly good for a healthy heart. Certain sulphur compounds found in garlic have the ability to lower cholesterol levels and prevent blood clots by reducing the stickiness of platelets (blood particles involved in the clotting process).

Garlic also plays an important role in protecting the respiratory system, helping to reduce mucus build-up and congestion. This is why it is valuable as a treatment for colds and flu and more serious respiratory disorders, such as bronchitis and whooping cough.

One of the key phytonutrients found in garlic, ajoene, is specifically antifungal. It encourages the growth of beneficial bacteria and has been shown to be effective against *Candida Albicans* as well as *Aspergillus niger* (fungi that can cause ear infections).

How to use garlic in your child's diet

To receive maximum benefit from garlic, you should add it at the end of cooking time. This prevents the heat from damaging its active ingredients. When garlic is crushed, it is best to let it stand for a few minutes to allow the enzymatic process that produces allicin to occur. Garlic is available in a dried form, but there is no doubt that fresh garlic is the cheapest and most effective form available.

To ensure that your children enjoy the beneficial effects of garlic, add it to your meals as often as you like. Introduce garlic to children as babies and they will love it for life. Garlic does have a strong flavour and, once past the age of two, children are more resistant to trying new flavours. Garlic is safe to introduce to a baby of six months, if added to a recipe in small amounts. For older children, add raw, crushed garlic to dressings and soups and include it in stir-fries and risottos. Garlic can also be made into delicious dips (see right) and added raw to dishes, such as pesto and hummus, without your children even noticing. Never apply garlic directly on to the skin or neat into a child's mouth, as it is very strong and can cause severe irritation.

IMMUNE PROFILE

★ **NEGLIGIBLE IN AMOUNTS USED**

▨ **AJOENE, ALLICIN, PHENOLIC COMPOUNDS, SAPONINS**

✓ **ANTIBACTERIAL, ANTICARCINOGENIC, ANTIFUNGAL, ANTIVIRAL, ANTITHROMBOTIC**

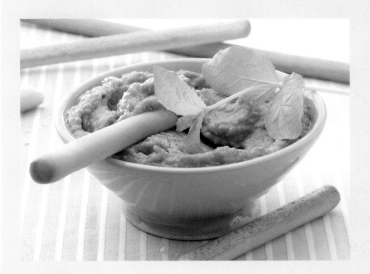

anchoiade

Depending on the amount of olive oil used, this makes an excellent dip or a tasty pasta sauce.

4 garlic cloves, peeled
1 packet of fresh anchovy fillets in olive oil and garlic
12 green olives, destoned
¼ cup (60 ml/2 fl oz) extra virgin olive oil
1 tsp balsamic vinegar

Put the garlic, anchovies and their oil and the green olives in a blender. Whizz up to form a paste. Add the balsamic vinegar and as much of the extra virgin olive oil as you require. This can either make a delicious dip or can be thinned to make a pasta sauce or dressing.

aioli

This creamy garlic mayonnaise makes a delicious dip or fine accompaniment to any salmon dish.

4 garlic cloves, peeled
2 egg yolks
2 tsp white wine vinegar
1 tsp lemon juice
½ tsp English mustard
⅜ cup (90 ml/3 fl oz) sunflower oil
⅜ cup (90 ml/3 fl oz) extra virgin olive oil

Place all the ingredients except the oils in a food processor. Blend the ingredients together and then very slowly drizzle the oil through the top of the food processor. This needs to take a long time as it is the gradual addition of the oil that causes the eggs to emulsify and all of the ingredients to thicken up.

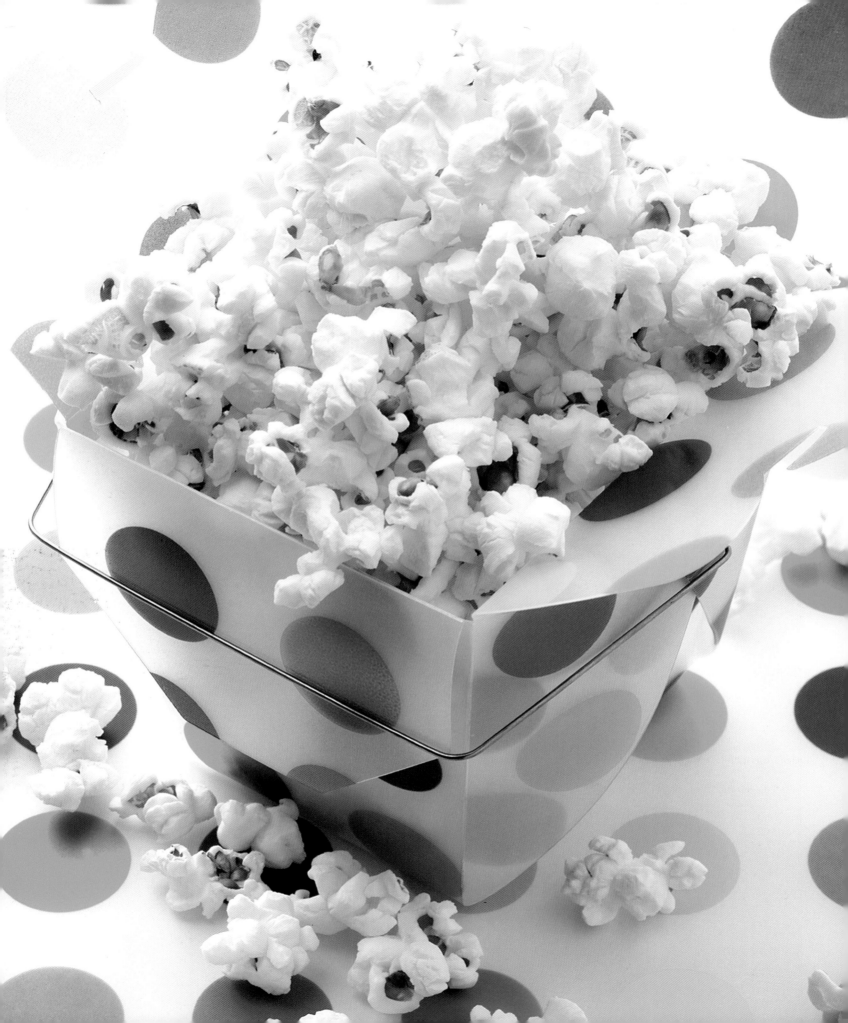

part three

immunity recipes for children

Whatever your child's age, the following pages will show you how to keep him healthy through diet. Whether you are weaning your baby or feeding teenagers, you will find mouthwatering recipes that are bursting with immune-boosting nutrients. The specific nutritional needs of children at each stage of their development are addressed and each age group has its own selection of recipes. Look out for the accompanying symbols, which include potential allergy information for each recipe. Units of measurement have been simplified wherever possible to enable quick and easy cooking. Hence you will find some ingredients measured by handfuls or pinches, and others by grammes. Metric, imperial and standard American cup units are used where appropriate. However, conversions are not exact, so keep to one set of measurements only when preparing a recipe. Feeding a family a healthy diet has never been easier.

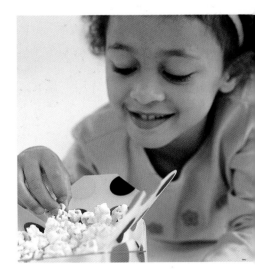

0–6 months

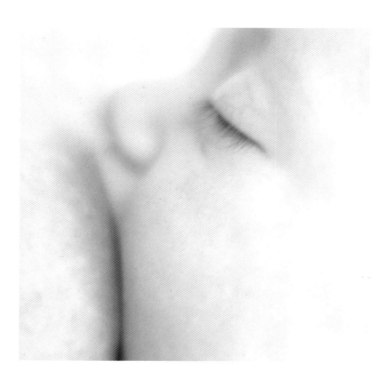

Your baby's immune system

Every baby is born with passive immunity (see page 10). This is the protection that the mother's immune system provides for her baby throughout pregnancy. At birth, your baby has a supply of maternal antibodies that helps protect him against the most common childhood infections, such as coughs, colds and chicken pox, in his first months. Prior to this, during the second and third trimesters of pregnancy, the baby's immune cells are forming, but they are not yet able to work on their own. It is not until the age of about six months that your baby's immune system can produce its own antibodies. This is good timing because the passively-acquired antibodies from the mother run out at around the same time.

Breastfeeding is best

During the first few months of your baby's life, breastfeeding is the best protection against illness and support for the baby's immune system that a mother can provide. Breast milk helps to ward off infections more common in bottle-fed babies, provides protection against allergies and will supply substances that can actively encourage your baby's immune system to develop. Many of these substances cannot be replicated in formula milks. Breast milk is particularly rich in IgA antibodies (see page 11), which line your baby's gut and protect against gastrointestinal infections.

Breast milk is a good source of highly absorbable minerals, antioxidants and other antibacterial substances that further help protect your baby against bacterial and viral infection. In addition, it contains enzymes that are protective against parasitic infections such as Giardia, which can cause diarrhoea in babies. Breast milk is also an excellent source of essential fatty acids. These are vital to the proper development and functioning of your child's immune system, as they help to regulate the activity of disease-fighting white blood cells and to protect your baby against allergies.

Eating for two

While you are breastfeeding, it is important to look after yourself. Feeding and caring for a new baby is very tiring so it helps to have lots of healthy, nutrient-packed snacks around to provide you with energy. Fruit smoothies, nut and seed bars, fruit, yoghurt and wholemeal sandwiches will all help to provide sustainable energy throughout the day. Other useful tips include the following:

• drink plenty of water. Your body needs more liquid to produce breast milk and avoiding additives commonly found in soft drinks will benefit both you and your baby.

• eat five portions of fruit and vegetables every day. This will provide the fibre, vitamins and phytonutrients needed by you and your baby. Making fresh vegetable and fruit juices each morning is a great way to supply both of you with an antioxidant boost.

• avoid taking stimulants while you are breastfeeding. Caffeine (found in coffee, tea, fizzy drinks and chocolate) can cause irritability and restlessness in both you and your baby. Other substances to avoid include alcohol, over-the-counter drugs, nicotine and artificial sweeteners, all of which can have a similarly detrimental effect on your baby.

SUGGESTED WEEKLY MENU PLANNER

	Monday	Tuesday	Wednesday	Thursday	Friday	Saturday	Sunday
breakfast	Crunchy Muesli (page 86) with sliced banana	Boiled eggs and toast, kiwi fruit	Protein Shake (page 62)	Porridge with Banana and Tahini (page 62)	Baked beans on toast, apple	Crunchy Muesli (page 86) with sliced banana	Poached egg and grilled tomato on toast
snack	Fruit	Fruit	Fruit	Fruit	Fruit	Fruit	Fruit
lunch	Handy Hummus with Baked Potato (page 74) with salad	Hearty Lentil Soup (page 62) with homemade bread	Sardine, Anchovy and Spinach Pâté (page 65) with crispbread	Pine Nut, Avocado, Red Onion and Watercress Salad Sandwich (page 65)	Watercress Soup and Walnut Bread (page 63)	Seafood Paella (page 66) with salad	Roast chicken and vegetables
snack	Ginger Cake (page 66), fruit	Fruit and Nut Bar (page 66), fruit	Almond butter on toast, fruit	Sesame and Honey bar (page 99), fruit	Yoghurt with banana and wheatgerm	Banana and Raisin Cake (page 83), fruit	Muesli Squares (page 83), fruit
supper	Venison Steaks with Butternut Squash and Cinnamon (page 63) with broccoli	Quick and Easy Seafood Pasta Supper (page 63) with crunchy salad	Chicken and Coconut Curry (page 64) with rice and salad	Warming Lentil and Potato Bake (page 64) with watercress salad	Pheasant Paysanne (page 79) with mashed potatoes and green beans	Coconut and Cauliflower Soup (page 63) with yeast-free bread	Roasted Vegetables with Coriander Couscous (page 65)

Protection for a bottle-fed baby

Perhaps because of illness or surgery, some women may not be able to breastfeed. Formula milks are the only option and there are many now available. If allergies run in the family, avoid cow's milk formulas, and opt for a goat's milk formula instead. Compare the essential fatty acid profile of the different formulas and choose one with good levels added. Once you have chosen, here are my tips:

• add a quarter of a teaspoon of an infant probiotic to your baby's bottle once a day, to provide some of the beneficial bacteria present in breast milk that help protect against gastrointestinal infection.

• add a few drops of organic linseed oil into each of your baby's bottles to provide a source of omega-3 essential fatty acids. Give a maximum of 1 teaspoon in 24 hours.

• rub the contents of a 500 mg evening primrose oil capsule onto your baby's tummy after bathtime to ensure a source of omega-6 essential fatty acids.

• don't overfeed your baby. This is common in bottle-fed babies. Stick to the number of bottles and the dilution suggested on the formula tin. Fat cells are laid down in infancy and an overweight baby is likely to become an overweight adult.

KISSING YOUR BABY – AN IMMUNE CONNECTION

Rather remarkably, breastfeeding mothers can protect their babies by providing tailor-made antibodies to the bacteria and viruses with which their baby comes into contact.

As a mother, you will already have a plethora of antibodies that have been created throughout your own life to protect you against certain diseases. Many of these diseases will be irrelevant to your newborn baby, but others will give a vital boost to his immune system. When you kiss your baby's cheek, you are effectively sampling the bacteria and viruses on his face that he is about to ingest. By transferring these bacteria to your own body, you stimulate your immune system to create specific antibodies to fight these pathogens (disease-causing microbes). You then pass the tailor-made antibodies back to your baby through your breast milk. What a miracle of nature!

breastfeeding recipes

Breastfeeding and coping with the demands of a very young baby can be thoroughly exhausting and the recipes in this section have been designed with this in mind. As well as being packed with energy and immune-boosting nutrients to benefit you and your baby, they are delicious and simple to prepare. All recipes serve two adults unless otherwise stated and all ingredients should be organic, where possible. The key to the recipe symbols can be found on page 5. The age-suitability for each recipe, both in Part Three and throughout the book, is based on the potential allergy risk of some of the ingredients and should be used in conjunction with your family's specific tastes and requirements.

BREAKFASTS

protein shake

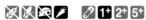

1 cup (225 ml/8 fl oz) apple juice
1 banana
1 tbsp linseed (flaxseed) oil
1 cup (225 g/8 oz) silken tofu
1 tsp molasses
1 tbsp wheatgerm

Liquidize all the ingredients and serve immediately.

porridge with banana, tahini, honey and soaked linseeds

 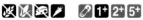

1 cup (100 g/3½ oz) porridge oats
water to cover
1 tbsp tahini
1 tbsp linseeds (flaxseeds), soaked
1 ripe banana
1 tbsp runny honey
A little soya milk (or milk if dairy-tolerant)

Put the oats and water in a saucepan and cook gently until the porridge has thickened. Take the pan off the heat, stir in the tahini and soaked linseeds and transfer the porridge to two pudding bowls. Slice the banana over the top and drizzle on the honey. Pour over a little soya milk or semi-skimmed milk.

MAIN MEALS

The first three recipes listed are soups that make great meals served with hunks of homemade bread. They are quick and easy, so are ideal to make when you are tired and having to cope with the demands of a new baby.

hearty lentil soup

 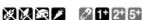

1 medium onion, chopped
1 garlic clove, chopped
1 tbsp extra virgin olive oil
1 tbsp medium curry powder
1 carrot, peeled and chopped
2 sticks celery, trimmed and chopped
600 ml (1 pint) vegetable stock
½ cup (100 g/3½ oz) red lentils
A handful of fresh coriander, chopped

Gently cook the onion and garlic in the olive oil until transparent. Add the curry powder and stir for 1 minute. Add the vegetables, the stock and the lentils. Bring to the boil, cover and gently simmer for 25 minutes until the vegetables are tender. Blend in a liquidizer and sprinkle with the coriander. Serve with Sesame Pitta Strips (see right).

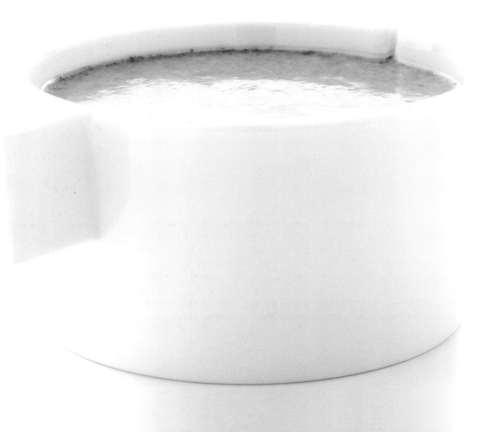

watercress soup *below left*

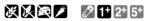

1 tbsp extra virgin olive oil
1 onion, chopped
2 medium potatoes, diced
A bunch of watercress, well washed
600 ml (1 pint) vegetable stock

Heat the oil gently in a large saucepan, add the onion and cook until transparent. Add the potatoes, watercress and the stock, cover and simmer for 20 minutes until the potatoes are soft. Once cooked, liquidize the soup and return it to the saucepan. Reheat gently and serve with Walnut Bread (see right).

coconut and cauliflower soup

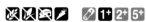

1 onion, chopped
1 garlic clove, crushed
1 tbsp extra virgin olive oil
1 small cauliflower, broken into florets
1 large carrot, chopped
1 tsp cumin seeds, ground
½ tsp turmeric
1 litre (1¾ pints) vegetable stock
1 tin of butter beans (no-sugar, no-salt variety)
¼ cup (60 g/2 oz) creamed coconut
A handful of fresh coriander, chopped

In a large saucepan, gently cook the onion and garlic in the olive oil. Add the cauliflower, carrot and spices and cook on a low heat for a couple of minutes, stirring all the time. Add the vegetable stock and the butter beans. Cover and simmer gently for 20 minutes until the cauliflower is soft. Add the coconut and stir until it has all melted. Serve sprinkled with fresh coriander.

quick and easy seafood pasta supper

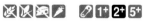

4 spring onions, chopped
1 tbsp extra virgin olive oil
1 small packet of smoked salmon
1 packet of frozen, cooked tiger prawns
A handful of uncooked wholemeal spaghetti
A couple of tbsps crème fraîche (optional)
A handful of chives

In a wok, gently stir-fry the spring onions in the olive oil for a couple of minutes until just cooked. Do not allow them to brown as this will change their flavour. When cooked, add the smoked salmon and the tiger prawns and stir well for a couple of minutes. Meanwhile, cook the wholemeal spaghetti. Once the spaghetti is ready, place it in a big serving bowl and stir in the fish mixture. If you wish to include the crème fraîche, stir it in at this stage. Finally, take a pair of kitchen scissors and snip the chives into little pieces over the top for extra flavour and a pretty, decorative effect.

sesame pitta strips

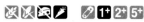

2 pitta breads
Olive oil for brushing
Sesame seeds for sprinkling

Preheat the oven to 200°C/400°F/Gas Mark 6. Brush the pitta bread on one side with some olive oil. Sprinkle with sesame seeds and cut into strips widthways. Place on a baking sheet and bake in the oven for 10 minutes.

walnut bread

 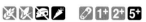

1 large onion, chopped
4 tbsp extra virgin olive oil
¼ cup (30 g/1¼ oz) pine nuts, plus some extra for sprinkling
⅓ cup (40 g/1½ oz) walnuts, chopped
450 g (1 lb) wholemeal flour
2 tsp cumin seeds
2 tsp coriander seeds
A handful of fresh coriander, chopped
1 tsp sea salt
300 ml (½ pint) warm filtered water
1 packet of easy blend dried yeast
Sesame seeds for sprinkling

In a saucepan, gently cook the onion in about half of the olive oil for a couple of minutes. Add the pine nuts and allow to brown slightly. Transfer to a mixing bowl and add the walnuts and the flour. Crush the cumin and coriander seeds in a pestle and mortar and add to the bowl. Stir in the chopped coriander and sea salt. Make a well in the centre of the flour mixture, pour in the water and sprinkle the yeast into the water. Mix together, then add the remainder of the olive oil to form a dough. Turn out onto a lightly floured surface and knead for 5 minutes. Put the dough back into the bowl and cover. Leave in a warm place for an hour to allow it to rise. After the hour, turn out the dough and mould it into a round shape on a lightly-oiled baking tray or place it in a lightly-oiled circular cake tin. Sprinkle with a few sesame seeds and pine nuts and bake in the oven at 200°C/400°F/Gas Mark 6 for 1 hour. Turn the bread out onto a rack and leave to cool.

venison steaks with baked butternut squash and cinnamon

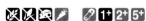

1 butternut squash
A sprinkling of cinnamon
2 venison steaks

Wash the butternut squash. Cut open lengthways, remove the seeds and cut into chunks, leaving the skin on. Place on a baking tray, flesh upwards, sprinkle with cinnamon and bake in the oven at 200°C/400°F/Gas Mark 6 for 45 minutes. Meanwhile, grill or griddle the venison for 8 minutes on each side or until cooked through. Serve with new potatoes and French beans.

chicken and coconut curry

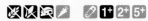

1 onion, chopped
1 tbsp extra virgin olive oil
3 bay leaves
2-inch piece of cinnamon stick
4 cloves
1 tsp coriander seeds, ground
1 tsp freshly grated ginger
½ tsp turmeric
2 chicken breasts, cut into small pieces
1 tin of chopped tomatoes
1 tbsp runny honey
½ tin of coconut milk

Gently sauté the onion in the olive oil. Add the herbs and spices and cook for a couple of minutes, stirring well. Add the chicken and cook for 3–4 minutes until the pieces have been sealed. Pour in the tomatoes, honey and coconut milk and simmer for around 15 minutes until the chicken is cooked through. Remove the bay leaves, cinnamon stick and cloves. Serve with brown rice, a green salad and a variety of chutneys and relishes.

warming lentil and potato bake

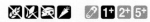

Cumin is a spice traditionally used to stimulate milk production in breastfeeding mothers.

1 medium onion, chopped
2 tbsp olive oil
1 garlic clove, crushed
1 tsp cumin seeds
1 tsp freshly grated ginger
2 medium potatoes, diced small
½ cup (115 g/4 oz) red lentils
600 ml (1 pint) vegetable stock
A handful of fresh coriander, chopped

In a large saucepan, gently cook the onion in the oil for 8–10 minutes. Add the garlic, cumin and ginger and stir to coat with the oil. Add the potatoes and stir again. Add the lentils and stock and bring to the boil. Cover and gently simmer for 25 minutes until the potatoes are cooked and the stock has all been absorbed. Sprinkle the coriander over the top and serve with a crunchy green salad.

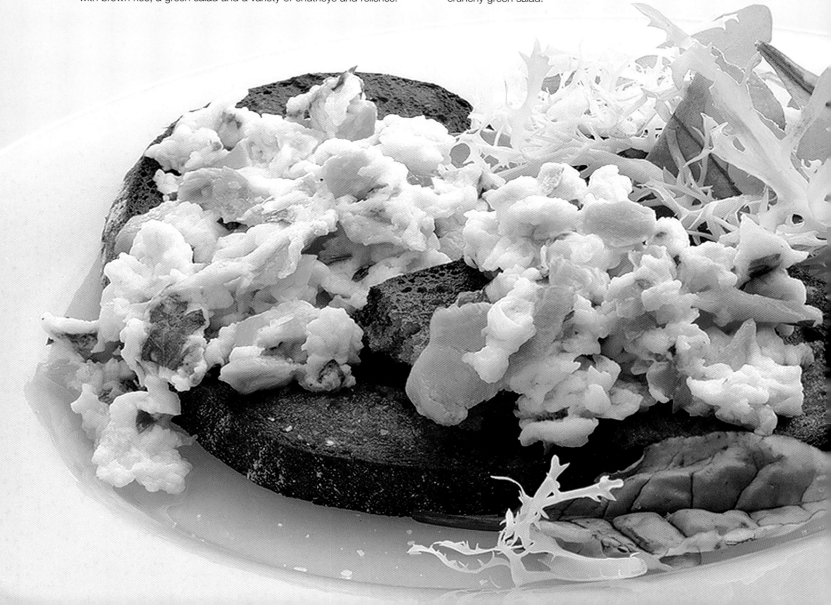

roasted vegetables with coriander couscous

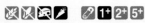 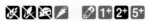

1 tbsp extra virgin olive oil
4 mini aubergines, halved
6 cherry tomatoes, halved
2 courgettes, chopped
4 garlic cloves, whole
2 garlic cloves, chopped
1 red onion, quartered lengthways
1 red pepper, deseeded and sliced
A handful of fresh basil, chopped
1 tbsp balsamic vinegar
500 g (1 lb 2 oz) ready-cooked couscous
600 ml (1 pint) vegetable stock
A handful of fresh coriander, chopped
2 handfuls of chopped walnuts, cashews, sunflower and pumpkin seeds, lightly roasted

Preheat the oven to 230°C/450°F/Gas Mark 8. Pour the olive oil into the bottom of a roasting pan. Add the vegetables and the basil. Toss the vegetables in the oil and add the vinegar. Bake in the preheated oven for 1 hour until brown around the edges. Soak the couscous in the vegetable stock for 5 minutes. Drain the couscous and put in a large flat serving dish. Add the chopped coriander to the couscous and pile the roasted vegetables on top. Sprinkle with the roasted nuts and seeds to serve.

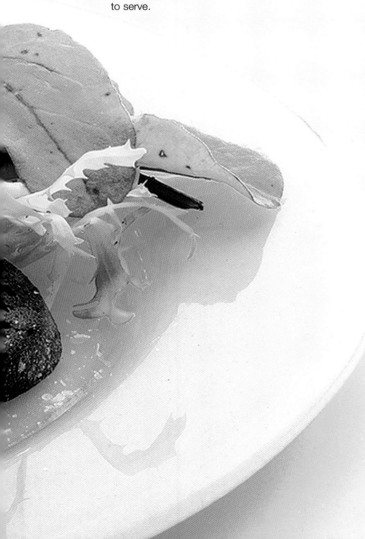

pine nut, avocado, red onion and watercress salad sandwich

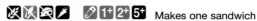   Makes one sandwich

This sandwich provides a good balance of protein, carbohydrate and essential fats for a breastfeeding mother.

A small handful of pine nuts, roasted
½ an avocado, sliced
A few slices of red onion
A couple of sprigs of watercress, roughly chopped
A splash of balsamic vinegar and olive oil, mixed together
2 slices rye bread, lightly buttered

Place the roasted pine nuts, avocado, onion and watercress in a bowl. Add the balsamic vinegar and olive oil and mix well. Transfer the mixture onto a lightly buttered piece of rye bread and top with another piece. Cut in half and eat immediately.

smoked salmon scramble *left*

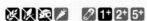

Instant food at its best.

4 eggs, beaten
A dash of soya milk (or semi-skimmed milk if dairy-tolerant)
1 small packet of smoked salmon, shredded
A handful of parsley
A knob of unhydrogenated vegetable margarine (or butter if dairy-tolerant)

In a glass jug, beat the eggs together with the soya milk, salmon and parsley. Melt some margarine in a non-stick saucepan. Pour in the egg mixture and cook over a low heat, stirring all the time. Once it has thickened, serve on wholemeal or rye toast with a handful of baby leaf salad and some dressing.

sardine, anchovy and spinach pâté

This iron-rich recipe can be made in advance and keeps for a couple of days in the fridge. Ideal for the demands of motherhood.

1 small onion, chopped
1 tbsp extra virgin olive oil
1 packet of baby leaf spinach
A sprig of fresh tarragon
A handful of parsley
4 fresh anchovy fillets in garlic
2 hard boiled eggs
1 tin of sardines in oil

In a saucepan, lightly cook the onion in the olive oil until transparent. Add the spinach, tarragon and parsley and allow the spinach to wilt. Place the contents of the pan in a food processor along with all of the other ingredients and blend until smooth. Put into the fridge for 30 minutes before eating. Serve with wholemeal toast and a crunchy salad.

seafood paella

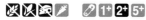

A 30-minute recipe, rich in iron, zinc and antioxidants.

1 onion, finely chopped
2 garlic cloves, crushed
1 green pepper, deseeded and diced
1 red pepper, deseeded and diced
2 tbsp extra virgin olive oil
A pinch of turmeric
4 squid tubes, cut into rings
2 handfuls of peeled prawns
1 monkfish tail, deboned and flesh cubed
2 plum tomatoes, skinned and chopped
1 cup (200 g/7 oz) long-grain brown rice or paella rice
600 ml (1 pint) vegetable stock
½ cup (100 g/3½ oz) frozen peas
A handful of parsley, chopped

In a paella pan or large flat frying pan, gently cook the onion, garlic and peppers in the olive oil until soft. Add the turmeric and cook for a further minute. Add the squid, prawns and monkfish and stir for a couple of minutes. Add the tomatoes and rice and cook for a further minute or two before adding all of the stock. Allow to bubble hard for a couple of minutes. Stir well, then simmer gently for 25 minutes until all the stock has been absorbed. In the last 10 minutes, scatter the peas over the paella. Once cooked, sprinkle with chopped parsley and serve direct from the pan with a large mixed salad.

PUDDINGS AND BAKING

ginger cake

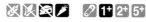

A hearty cake, rich in iron for breastfeeding mothers.

½ cup (60 g/2 oz) wholemeal flour
½ cup (90 g/3 oz) oatmeal
2 tsp baking powder
2 tsp ground ginger
¼ cup (90 g/3 oz) molasses
¼ cup (60 g/2 oz) fructose
¼ cup (115 ml/4 fl oz) sunflower oil or extra virgin olive oil
¼ cup (115 ml/4 fl oz) water
2 eggs, beaten
¼ cup (30 g/1 oz) flaked almonds

Preheat the oven to 180°C/350°F/Gas Mark 4. In a bowl, mix together the flour, oatmeal, baking powder and ginger. Gently heat the molasses, fructose and oil together until blended. Add the water and pour into the dry ingredients along with the beaten eggs. Mix well and pour into a well-greased rectangular bread tin. Sprinkle with the almonds and bake for 30 minutes until the mixture is well-risen and a knife comes out clean when pushed into the centre of the cake. Turn out and cool on a wire rack.

summer fruits brulée *right*

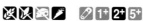

4 large strawberries
2 tbsp blueberries
2 tbsp raspberries
4 tbsp thick and creamy natural yoghurt
2 tbsp dark muscovado sugar

Separate the fruit into two ramekin-type dishes in equal amounts. Add a couple of spoonfuls of yoghurt to each dish and top with a tablespoon of sprinkled sugar. Place under a hot grill until the sugar bubbles.

fruit and nut bars

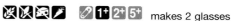 makes 12–15 bars

These make an excellent snack at any time of day.

½ cup (115 g/4 oz) unhydrogenated vegetable margarine (or butter if dairy-tolerant)
½ cup (115 ml/4 fl oz) apple juice concentrate
½ cup (75 g/3 oz) mixed dried fruit
½ cup (90 g/3 oz) porridge oats
½ cup (60 g/2 oz) chopped mixed nuts
½ cup (60 g/2 oz) wholemeal flour

Preheat the oven to 180°C/350°F/Gas Mark 4. In a saucepan, melt the margarine and the apple juice concentrate together. Add all of the other ingredients and mix well. Spoon the mixture into a lightly-greased, shallow square tin and press down hard. Bake for 20–25 minutes until golden brown. Cut the bars in the tin and leave to cool before removing. Store in an airtight container.

DRINK

mint and mango smoothie

 makes 2 glasses

Refreshing, and rich in beta-carotene and vitamin C. Including mint in the diet of a breastfeeding mother can give relief to a colicky baby as it is very calming to the digestive tract.

6 ice cubes, crushed
2 kiwi fruit, peeled
1 mango, peeled and chopped
A handful of mint
1 cup (225 ml/8 fl oz) filtered water

Put all the ingredients into a blender or food processor and whizz together. Serve immediately.

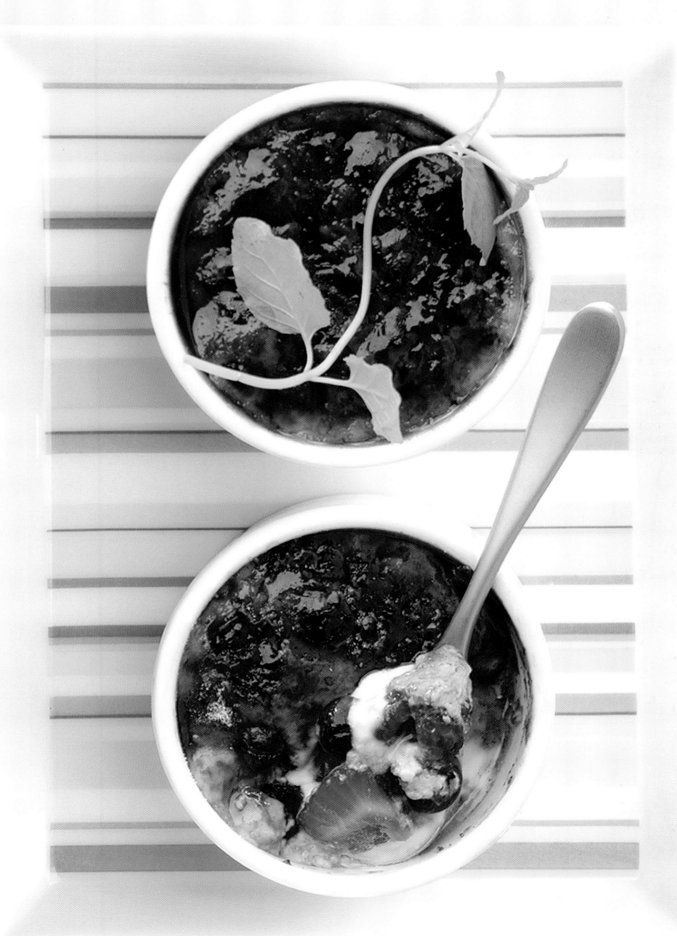

6–12 months

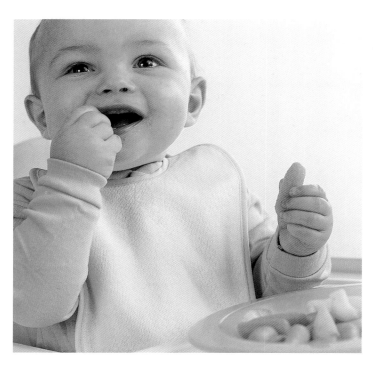

Immune-boosting weaning for your baby

At around the age of six months your baby will be ready for solid food. It is at this time that the passively acquired antibodies he received in the womb will have run out. He will have encountered numerous germs in the environment and his immune system will be starting to create its own antibodies to provide some protection against infection. Delaying weaning until the age of six months has several benefits for your baby. As the immune system will have had that crucial bit longer to develop, it is less susceptible to becoming sensitized against certain foods, so your baby will have a reduced risk of developing allergies. This is particularly important where there is a family history of allergy, such as asthma, eczema, migraine or hay fever. Also, avoiding introducing solids before six months helps prevent unnecessary strain being placed on an immature digestive system. However, it is important not to leave the introduction of solids until much later than six months as your baby's iron stores from birth will be running low by this time.

How you introduce your baby to solids is as important as when you choose to do it. You need to gradually introduce a range of fruits, vegetables, grains and proteins so that your child's immune system can maximize the nutritional benefits of his diet at this critical time. I suggest you follow the weaning chart opposite, along with the Protecting Babies Against Allergies chart (see page 115) for the best immune-boosting weaning plan for your child.

All you need for weaning, in practical terms, are a few plastic spoons and a small weaning bowl. Begin by giving your baby tiny tastes of fruit and vegetable purées, one food at a time so that you can see if there is any reaction to a particular food. Introduce solid food first at lunchtime and offer it in the middle of a milk feed so your baby will not be so hungry that he will dismiss the food and cry only for milk, nor will he be too full to take any notice of it at all.

Once your baby has tried a variety of fruits and vegetables, start to blend the flavours and introduce grains and protein foods. By the age of seven months, he should be on three meals a day, and by nine months solid food will be taking over from the milk feeds with these becoming top-ups at the end of a meal. However, a baby still needs 600 ml (1 pint) of breast milk or formula a day up until the age of one. This is the equivalent of two large bottles or two good breast milk feeds and includes any milk added to food.

While weaning a baby onto solid food, cook purées in bulk, freeze them in ice-cube trays and then transfer them into plastic freezer bags. This prevents unnecessary waste and, as the variety of his diet expands, you can mix and match any leftovers. In addition, some fruits and vegetables, such as banana, avocado, papaya, melon, mango and soft ripe pear, can be served raw. Raw foods retain all the vitamins and minerals lost during cooking and it is good to develop a baby's taste for them.

Ideally, first foods should be organic and as fresh as possible. Weight for weight, babies consume far more fruits and vegetables than adults, so their pesticide exposure from non-organic products will be far higher at a time when they are most vulnerable. Even if you never use organic foods again, use them now to protect your baby from these chemicals, which are known to be carcinogenic.

FOUR-WEEK WEANING CHART

Here is a guide to weaning your baby onto solid food. All babies vary so if your baby wants to eat more than is suggested that is fine. Also, if you choose to start your baby on solid food before the age of 6 months, this chart still applies. Introduce a beaker of water around the age of 6 months at mealtimes. Most babies take some time to get used to using a beaker, but will have mastered the technique between 8 and 10 months.

		week 1	week 2	week 3	week 4
breakfast				up to 2 cubes of a cereal and fruit purée in middle of the milk feed	up to 3 cubes of a cereal and fruit purée in middle of the milk feed
lunch		up to 1 cube of a single fruit or vegetable purée in middle of the milk feed	up to 2 cubes of a single fruit or vegetable purée in middle of the milk feed	up to 3 cubes of a double fruit or vegetable purée before the milk feed	up to 3 cubes of a double vegetable purée followed by fruit purée before the milk feed
supper					up to 2 cubes of a double fruit or vegetable purée before the milk feed

SUGGESTED WEEKLY MENU PLANNER

		Monday	Tuesday	Wednesday	Thursday	Friday	Saturday	Sunday
6 MONTHS	lunch	My First Carrot Purée (page 70)	My First Carrot Purée (page 70)	Apple purée	Apple purée	Butternut squash purée	Butternut squash purée	Avocado purée
8 MONTHS	breakfast	Millet Porridge with Date Purée (page 72)	Baby rice with apple purée	Millet Porridge (page 72) with Dried Apricot Purée (page 75)	Oat porridge with pear purée	Brown rice purée with banana purée	Millet Porridge (page 72) with papaya purée	Oat porridge with apple and molasses purée
	lunch	Vegetable Medley (page 70)	Chicken Casserole (page 72)	Immune-boosting Lentil Purée (page 73)	Cod and Veggies (page 73)	Avocado and Banana Purée (page 70)	My First Fish Pie (page 74)	Vegetable Medley (page 70)
	supper	Vegetable or fruit combo purée	Vegetable or fruit combo purée	Vegetable or fruit combo purée	Vegetable or fruit combo purée	Vegetable or fruit combo purée	Vegetable or fruit combo purée	Vegetable or fruit combo purée
10 MONTHS	breakfast	My First Muesli (page 72)	Millet Porridge (page 72) with fruit purée	Baby muesli	Brown rice purée and banana	Vegetable or fruit combo purée	Millet Porridge (page 72) with papaya purée	My First Muesli (page 72)
	lunch	Sweet Potato and Tahini (page 74), fruit purée	Venison Shepherd's Pie (page 74) with broccoli	Handy Hummus with Baked Potato (page 74), fruit purée	My First Fish Pie (page 74), fruit purée	Tempting Tofu Pasta Sauce (page 74) with rice pasta spirals	My First Pasta Sauce (page 73) with corn pasta, fruit purée	Roast chicken and vegetables, fruit purée
	supper	My First Pasta Sauce (page 73) with corn pasta, apple purée and date purée	Fruit purée, Vegetable Medley (page 70), banana pieces	Immune-boosting Lentil Purée (page 73) with buckwheat pasta, Dried Apricot Purée (page 75)	Vegetable combo purée, semolina with fruit purée	Fruit purée, avocado, banana and sprouted seed purée	Cod and Veggies (page 73), mango and banana purée	Vegetable Medley (page 70), Baked Apple with Raisins and Spices (page 75)

6–12 months recipes

This section includes recipes that are suitable as first weaning foods, as well as recipes that are designed for older babies with more adventurous appetites. All ingredients should be organic wherever possible to avoid potentially harmful pesticide residues. Cross refer with the Menu Planner (page 69), and the Protecting Babies Against Allergies chart (page 115) to check which foods are ideally suited to your baby's current age. There are many other recipes you can cook to provide variety for your baby. Some recipes elsewhere in the book can also be given to young babies so look out for the codes. Note: for the purées, the different recipes produce differing amounts of purée depending on the types of ingredients used but I have given an approximate guide to quantity, measured in ice-cube sized portions, for each one.

FIRST FRUIT AND VEGETABLE PURÉES

my first carrot purée

  makes approximately 24 cubes

Naturally sweet, carrot purée is ideal as a first food for a baby. It is rich in beta-carotene and other nutrients to help protect your baby against infection.

1 bag of carrots
Filtered water for steaming

Wash, peel and chop the carrots and place in a steamer. Steam until they are really tender and then blend in a food processor with some of the cooking water to create a smooth and fairly runny purée.

butternut squash and broccoli purée

  makes approximately 42 cubes

Rich in antioxidants, this will help to strengthen your baby's immune system.

1 butternut squash
1 head of broccoli
Filtered water for steaming

Peel, deseed and chop up the squash. Wash and chop up the broccoli. Steam the vegetables together until soft. Purée and freeze in ice-cube trays.

vegetable medley

  makes approximately 54 cubes

A delicious blend of vegetables for a strong immune system.

1 head of broccoli
2 carrots
A handful of green beans
3 sweet potatoes
Filtered water for steaming

Steam the vegetables until tender. Blend in a food processor with 4 or 5 tablespoons of water from the steamer. Freeze in ice-cube portions or individual pots depending on your baby's appetite.

vegetable combos

 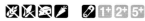

Combine different coloured and textured vegetables to create your own delicious vegetable bases. Experimentation is all part of the fun when you are preparing your own baby food. The following are some suggestions that you and your baby may like to try.

Carrot, kale, green bean and sweetcorn
Pumpkin, spinach and potato (suitable from 9 months)
Sweet potato, watercress and broccoli
Cauliflower, butternut squash, onion and celeriac
Beetroot, carrot, parsley and potato (suitable from 9 months)
Courgette, sweet potato and green cabbage
Carrot, parsnip and potato (suitable from 9 months)

avocado and banana purée

  makes 1 generous portion

Instant baby food at its best. Make sure that the banana is really ripe as unripe bananas can cause tummy aches and constipation. Banana and avocado are not easily frozen, so this is a purée that must be eaten straightaway.

½ ripe avocado
1 small ripe banana

Scoop out the flesh of the avocado and mash together with the banana. Serve straightaway.

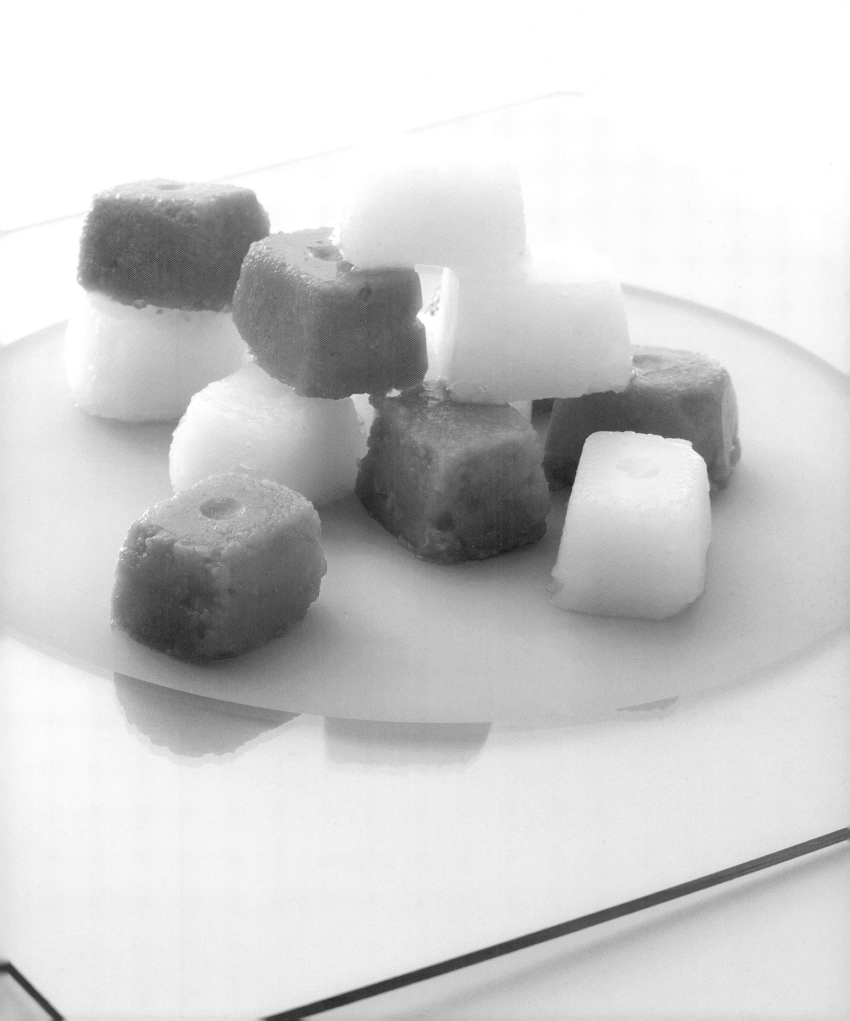

stewed apple purée with cloves and molasses

  makes approximately 28 cubes

All babies love apple purée and the molasses in this recipe adds an iron boost. Molasses has a strong and distinctive flavour, so do not be tempted to add more than the suggested amount.

1 bag of eating apples
1 cup (225 ml/8 fl oz) filtered water
1 clove
1 level tsp molasses

Peel and core the apples. Place in a saucepan with the water and the clove. Bring to the boil and simmer gently until soft. Once cooked, remove the clove and stir in the molasses. Purée and freeze in ice-cube trays.

date purée

 makes approximately 15 cubes

1 cup (225 ml/8 fl oz) filtered water
1 packet (250 g/9 oz) pitted dates (not sugar rolled)

Put the water and dates in a saucepan. Bring to the boil and gently simmer for 10 minutes until the dates have softened. While the dates are simmering, use a wooden spoon to break them up to form a mush. Blend the dates with any remaining water to form a smooth purée. Once cooled, spoon into a lidded glass jar and put in the fridge. This purée can be frozen or will keep fresh for two weeks if refrigerated.

FIRST CEREALS

millet porridge

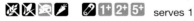 serves 1

Millet is rich in iron and easily digested. This quick and easy porridge is an ideal first grain for your baby.

1 tbsp ground millet flakes
150 ml (5 fl oz) breast milk, formula or filtered water

Using a non-stick saucepan, gently mix the millet with a little of the milk or water to form a paste and bring to the boil. Simmer gently, stirring all the time, until it thickens up. Add a little more milk for your desired consistency if it becomes too thick. Serve with a teaspoon of Date Purée (see above).

my first muesli

 from 8–9 months; serves 1

This muesli recipe is rich in omega-3 essential fatty acids, which are vital nutrients for a healthy immune system.

1 tbsp porridge oats
2 tbsp filtered water
½ ripe banana
1 tsp ground almonds
1 tsp linseed (flaxseed) oil

Soak the oats in the water overnight in the fridge. In the morning, add the banana, almonds and linseed oil. Purée or mash to your desired consistency.

FIRST PROTEIN PURÉES

chicken casserole

 makes approximately 40 cubes

This purée is packed full of vegetables rich in antioxidants.

2 skinless chicken thighs
6 baby carrots
6 baby corn
6 baby courgettes, topped and tailed
3 baby parsnips, peeled
2 spring onions, sliced (white part only)
A pinch of oregano
300 ml (½ pint) vegetable stock

Preheat the oven to 190°C/375°F/Gas Mark 5. Place the chicken thighs in a glass casserole dish and cover them with all of the vegetables and the oregano. Pour over the vegetable stock and bake for 35–40 minutes until the chicken is cooked through and falls off the bone. Once cooked, remove the bones from the chicken and purée or mash to your desired consistency.

vegetable stock

 makes 1 litre (1¾ pints)

This versatile homemade stock is rich in immune-boosting herbs.

5 shallots, peeled and chopped
1 garlic clove, crushed
2 tbsp olive oil
1 bay leaf
1 large carrot, peeled and chopped
1 stick celery, peeled and chopped
1 thin slice root ginger
1 sprig of fresh thyme
850 ml (1½ pints) filtered water

Gently cook the shallots and garlic in the olive oil. Add the rest of the ingredients and cover with the water. Bring to the boil, cover and gently simmer for 1 hour. Remove the bay leaf, ginger and thyme before liquidizing the stock and freezing in ice-cube trays.

immune-boosting lentil purée *below right*

  makes approximately 20 cubes

Red lentils are a useful source of iron for young babies.

1 tbsp extra virgin olive oil
1 medium onion, peeled and chopped
1 garlic clove, crushed
1 stick celery, trimmed and chopped
1 large carrot, peeled and chopped
A pinch of ground coriander
A pinch of ground ginger
2 heaped tbsp red lentils
1 cup (225 ml/8 fl oz) filtered water
1 tsp chopped parsley

Heat the oil in a saucepan and gently soften the onion, garlic, celery and carrot. Add the spices and the lentils and stir to coat the lentils with the oil. Add the water and simmer for 15 minutes until the lentils are soft. Once cooked, sprinkle the parsley over the mixture and mash or purée to your desired consistency.

cod and veggies

makes approximately 24 cubes

1 small onion, peeled and chopped
1 tbsp olive oil
1 small skinless and boneless cod fillet, diced
A handful of kale, stripped
A handful of millet grains, washed
1 small sweet potato, diced
1 cup (225 ml/8 fl oz) homemade vegetable stock or
   low-salt vegetable bouillon

In a saucepan, gently cook the onion in the olive oil. Add the cod fillet and cook for 3–4 minutes, stirring constantly. Add the rest of the ingredients, cover and simmer gently for 15–20 minutes until the vegetables and millet are soft. Purée to desired consistency.

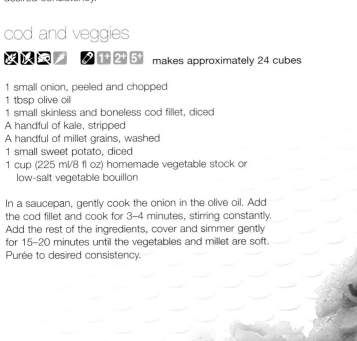

my first pasta sauce

  From 9 months; makes approximately 55 cubes

This dairy-free pasta sauce is packed with protein and immune-boosting nutrients. Tomatoes can provoke allergic reactions and should therefore be introduced to babies a little later than other vegetables.

2 onions, peeled and chopped
2 tbsp extra virgin olive oil
1 carrot, peeled and chopped
1 medium courgette, chopped
1 tin of flageolot beans (no-sugar, no-salt variety)
1 garlic clove, crushed
1 tin of chopped tomatoes (no-sugar, no-salt variety)
½ cup (100 ml/3½ fl oz) water
1 tbsp chopped basil

Gently cook the onion in the olive oil until translucent. Add all of the remaining ingredients except the basil and gently simmer for approximately 20 minutes until the vegetables are soft. Once cooked, add the basil and blend in a food processor to create a smooth sauce. Freeze as ice cubes or in small pots. Serve with rice pasta, buckwheat pasta or corn pasta. Today, a wide variety of wheat alternatives are available in health food shops and some supermarkets.

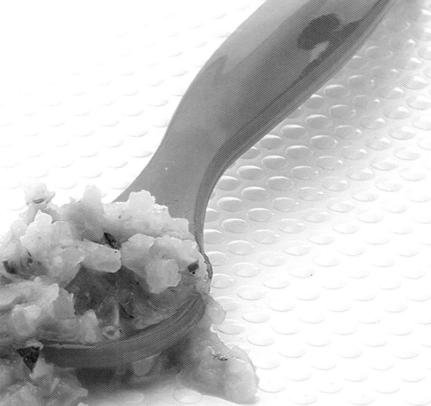

tempting tofu pasta sauce

 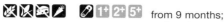   from 9 months;
makes 4 ramekin-size pots

This is a pasta sauce that can be enjoyed by vegetarians, vegans or meat-eating babies.

1 garlic clove, crushed
1 onion, peeled and chopped
2 tbsp extra virgin olive oil
A handful of shiitake mushrooms, chopped
1 tin of chopped tomatoes (no-sugar, no-salt variety)
½ pack of silken tofu, cubed

Gently cook the garlic and onion in the olive oil until translucent. Add the shiitake mushrooms and cook for a couple of minutes. Add the tomatoes and tofu and simmer for 10 minutes until the mushrooms are cooked through. Blend in a food processor to create a smooth sauce. Add some water if the end result is too thick. Serve with buckwheat or rice pasta. Freeze excess in ice-cube trays or small pots.

my first fish pie

 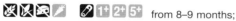   from 8–9 months;
makes 5 ramekin-size pots

These pies can be enjoyed by schoolchildren as well as babies. They are an excellent way of introducing oily fish to your family.

2 medium potatoes, peeled and chopped
1 onion, finely chopped
2 tbsp extra virgin olive oil
1 salmon fillet, chopped
1 tin of sweetcorn (no-sugar, no-salt variety)
1 small head of broccoli
6–8 cubes vegetable stock (page 72)

Cover the potatoes with water, bring to the boil and cook until tender. Then mash and put to one side. Gently cook the onions in the olive oil until transparent. Add the salmon and stir for a couple of minutes. Add the sweetcorn, broccoli and the cubes of vegetable stock. Cover the pan and simmer gently until the broccoli is tender and the fish is cooked through. Once cooked, transfer the salmon mixture into small pots and cover with the mashed potato. Serve immediately and freeze any additional portions.

handy hummus with baked potato

 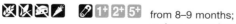   from 8–9 months;
makes approximately 40 cubes

A delicious hummus for all the family to enjoy.

1 baking potato
1 tin of chickpeas (no-sugar, no-salt variety)
1 garlic clove
Juice of ½ a lemon
10 tbsp extra virgin olive oil
A few sprigs of fresh parsley
1 tbsp tahini paste

Place all the ingredients, except the potato, together in a food processor and blend to form a smooth paste. Add a little more oil if the mixture appears too thick. Once made, you can store the hummus in the fridge for 2–3 days. Bake the potato in a moderate oven (190°C/375°F/Gas Mark 5) for 1 hour or until it is soft in the middle. Scoop out the flesh and mix with a teaspoon of hummus. You can also add some finely grated raw carrot or a slice of avocado for variety.

sweet potato and tahini

     from 9 months; serves 1

1 sweet potato
1 tsp tahini paste

Bake the sweet potato in a moderate oven (190°C/375°F/Gas Mark 5) for 35–40 minutes until soft. Scoop out the flesh into a bowl and mix with the tahini paste.

venison shepherd's pie

 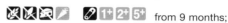   from 9 months;
makes 8 ramekin-size pots

Venison is low in saturated fat and rich in iron – a powerful combination to boost your baby's immune system.

1 onion, peeled and chopped
1 garlic clove, crushed
1 tbsp extra virgin olive oil
450 g (1 lb) venison mince
1 carrot, peeled and diced
1 courgette, diced
1 tin of chopped tomatoes (no-sugar, no-salt variety)
2 tbsp tomato purée
½ cup (115 ml/4 fl oz) vegetable stock
4 medium potatoes, peeled and quartered
A knob of vegetable margarine (or butter if dairy-tolerant)

In a saucepan, gently cook the onion and the garlic in the olive oil. Add the mince and brown well. Add the rest of the ingredients, except the potatoes. Stir well while bringing to the boil. Once boiling, turn down the heat and simmer gently for 1 hour, stirring occasionally. Meanwhile, boil the potatoes for 20–25 minutes and, once cooked, mash with a little margarine or butter. Pour the mince mixture into individual ramekin dishes or plastic freezer pots and cover with mashed potato.

PUDDINGS

semolina fruit pudding with dried apricot purée

  from 9–10 months; serves 1

Semolina is a good introduction to wheat. As wheat has allergic potential, this should only be an occasional pudding for babies.

2 tsp wholegrain semolina
150 ml (5 fl oz) breast milk, formula or fortified soya milk
1 cube dried apricot purée

Put the semolina in a saucepan and slowly add the milk, a little at a time to prevent lumps from forming. Gently simmer the semolina until it begins to thicken, but do not let it boil. Once it has thickened, remove from the heat and add a cube of dried apricot purée.

DRIED APRICOT PURÉE
Put the contents of a packet of unsulphured dried apricots in a pan and just cover them with water. Bring to the boil and gently simmer until they are very tender. Blend the apricots and the cooking water to a smooth purée and freeze in ice-cube trays.

baked apple with raisins and spices

   makes one serving

The molasses and raisins provide a useful source of iron for your baby.

1 eating apple, cored
1 tbsp raisins
1 level tsp molasses
A tiny pinch of cinnamon (optional)
A tiny pinch of ground cloves (optional)
6 tbsp water

Place the apple in a glass ovenware dish. In a separate bowl, mix the raisins, molasses, cinnamon and cloves. Fill the centre of the apple with the raisin mixture and surround the apple with the water. Bake in a moderate oven (190°C/375°F/Gas Mark 5) for 30–40 minutes, or until the apple is really soft. Scoop out the flesh of the apple and blend with the raisin mixture.

fruit smoothie pudding *below*

 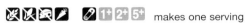 makes one serving

Any fruit can be added to a banana to make a delicious fruit purée pudding rich in antioxidants. Remember, however, to check the Protecting Babies Against Allergies chart (page 115) so you can choose a fruit that is suitable for your child's age.

1 banana
½ mango

In a food processor or liquidizer, blend the banana and mango to form a thick smoothie pudding.

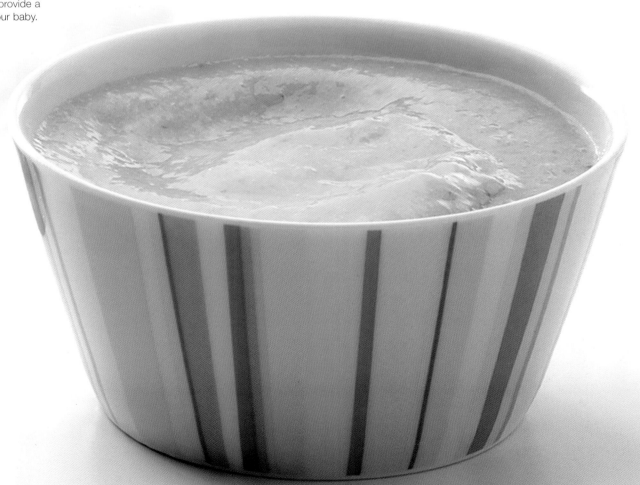

1–4 years

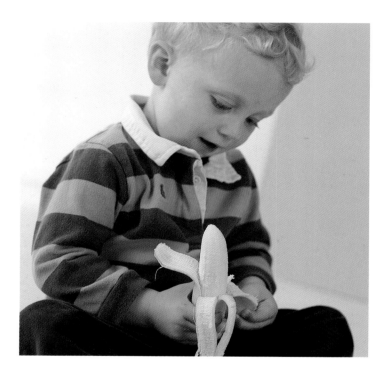

Nutritional needs of the pre-school child

From the age of one, your child should be eating more or less the same food as the rest of the family. He should have three meals a day and two snacks. Where possible, mealtimes should be family occasions, when you sit, eat and talk with your toddler. This is essential to build up good eating habits from an early age. A child with a parent who never sits down at a table or who is constantly on a diet and eating different food is likely to mimic this behaviour. If you want your child to eat well and be healthy then you need to do so, too! Obesity is becoming a serious problem in young children in the developed world, with as many as one in ten toddlers who are clinically obese. This is a condition directly linked to poor diet and can lead to all sorts of health problems, such as diabetes.

During the pre-school years, every parent needs to pay particular attention to his or her toddler's intake of certain nutrients. The most important nutrients to include are calcium, iron, magnesium, zinc, essential fatty acids and antioxidants, all of which generally help build up the immune system and promote growth and development. For explanations of the functions of each nutrient and examples of rich food sources, see the Essential Nutrients chart (pages 138–9).

Snacks for this age group should consist of fruit, fruit and seed bars, and homemade sugar-free cakes and biscuits, such as Banana and Raisin Cake (see page 83). Avoid sugary foods, which suppress immune activity and encourage poor eating habits as well as damaging baby teeth at a time when they are just appearing. Sweets and chocolate are party food not everyday food!

Encourage your toddler to drink water with meals rather than sugary squashes and fruit drinks, as these are often laden with sweeteners, colours and preservatives, which only increase the chemical burden on an immature immune system. Diluted fresh fruit juices or fruit smoothies are a far healthier alternative. Once a child reaches the age of one, milk or dairy-free milk alternatives should be regarded as food. Avoid giving them at mealtimes as they are very filling and your child may not want the rest of the meal. Instead, offer milk before breakfast or bed, or as a snack. Avoid fizzy drinks for this age group as they leach calcium from your child's body.

Your toddler's immune system

During the pre-school years, your toddler will be exposed to many different bacteria and viruses and each encounter will strengthen his immune defences. Most toddlers catch bugs from their siblings or other children. This is quite normal and an important part of the maturation of their immune systems. It is not normal, however, for these bugs to drag on. A child with a strong immune system will recover from a cold or other viral infection in two to three days. If your toddler seems constantly to be ill, you need to look at ways of further supporting his immune system through this period of his life.

In addition to bacterial or viral infection, stress can suppress a child's immune system, even at this young age. Signs of stress in a pre-school child might be incontinence, aggressive behaviour and night terrors. A stressed child may also be underweight. Stress hormones act as immuno-suppressants, resulting in more frequent infections. If you think that your child may be suffering from stress, consult your doctor.

SUGGESTED WEEKLY MENU PLANNER

	Monday	Tuesday	Wednesday	Thursday	Friday	Saturday	Sunday
breakfast	Parsley Eggs (page 78) with toast, tangerine	Fruity Scotch Pancakes (page 78) with mashed banana	My First Muesli (page 72), rice cakes with fruit spread	Almond butter on toast, Strawberry Smoothie (page 83)	Porridge with Banana, Tahini, Honey and Soaked Linseeds (page 62)	Creamy Cashew Porridge (page 78), pear slices	My First Muesli (page 72) with banana, toast soldiers
snack	Fruit, slice of Banana and Raisin Cake (page 83)	Fruit, Muesli Square (page 83)	Fruit, rice cakes with cashew butter	Fruit, Homemade Digestive Biscuits (page 91)	Fruit, fruit bar	Fruit, grissini sticks with hummus	Fruit, Popcorn (page 90)
lunch	Farmhouse Lentil Pie (page 82), Mango Hedgehog (page 83)	Venison Shepherd's Pie (page 74) with broccoli, Design a Bug (page 82)	Toddler Fish Pie (page 79) with French beans, banana custard	Turkey and Cranberry Burgers (page 79), Fruit Smoothie Pudding (page 75)	Pheasant Paysanne (page 79), Dairy-free Ice Cream (page 83)	Tuna Fishcakes (page 79), melon slices	Roast chicken with vegetables, baked apple and custard
snack	Fruit	Fruit	Fruit	Fruit	Fruit	Fruit	Fruit
supper	Rice pasta with My First Pasta Sauce (page 73), Homemade Yoghurt with Help Yourself Toppings (page 82)	Sweetcorn Patties (page 81) with green salad, Homemade Yoghurt with Four Fruit Purée (page 51)	Handy Hummus with Baked Potato (page 74) with salad sticks, 100% Fruit Jam Tarts (page 90)	Quick and Easy Beany Bake (page 80) with salad, yoghurt or Homemade Soya Yoghurt (page 51)	Make Your Own Pizza (page 80), pear and apple slices	Pasta with Tempting Tofu Pasta Sauce (page 74) with cucumber slices, Muesli Square (page 83)	Picnic or sandwich tea

Does my toddler need to eat dairy products?

Dairy products are a good source of protein, carbohydrate, fat, calcium and fat-soluble vitamins, and have become a staple part of our diet in the West. However, many cultures do not eat dairy products at all and seem to thrive quite happily without them. Indeed, with the rise of allergic conditions, such as eczema and asthma, and other complaints, including childhood diabetes, in children in the West, some healthcare professionals are questioning the role that dairy products play in our children's diets.

Calcium is probably the key nutrient with which we associate dairy products, but children do not have to eat dairy to get enough of it. Plenty of other foods are valuable calcium sources, and many of these are also rich in magnesium, which is required for proper calcium utilization. A child needs 350 mg of calcium a day between the ages of one and three years and 450 mg between the ages of four and six years. Look at the chart, right, and you will see how easy it is to achieve this level of calcium without dairy products.

CALCIUM IN FOOD

FOOD (100 g/ml)	CALCIUM (mg)
Whole cow's milk	115
Calcium-enriched soya milk	140
Calcium-enriched rice milk	120
Cheddar cheese	720
Natural yoghurt	200
Calcium-enriched soya yoghurt	100
Calcium-enriched tofu	150
Watercress	170
Spinach (cooked)	160
Kale (cooked)	150
Sardines (in oil)	550
Prawns	150
Tahini paste	680
Almonds	240
Molasses (one tablespoon)	140

1–4 years recipes

Now that your toddler can eat the same meals as the rest of the family, these recipes are designed to feed two adults and two children unless otherwise stated in the recipe itself. All ingredients should be organic, where possible, to protect young immune systems.

BREAKFASTS

fruity scotch pancakes

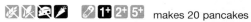 makes 20 pancakes

3 eggs, separated
1 cup (115 g/4 oz) wholemeal flour
1 tsp baking powder
1 tsp cream of tartar
1 cup (225 ml/8 fl oz) soya milk (or whole milk if dairy-tolerant)
1 cup (150 g/5½ oz) sun-dried raisins

In a mixing bowl, place the egg yolks, flour, baking powder, cream of tartar and milk and mix together well. Whisk the egg whites until they form peaks. Add them to the mixing bowl. Sprinkle over the raisins. Fold all of the ingredients together. Heat a non-stick frying pan and when really hot add tablespoonfuls of the batter to form small pancakes. When bubbles appear on the top of the pancakes, flip them over and cook for a further minute or so on the other side. Serve with mashed bananas.

creamy cashew porridge

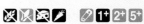

2 cups (200 g/7 oz) porridge oats
Filtered water to cover
A handful of cashew nuts, finely ground
2 tbsp linseed (flaxseed) oil
Runny honey or molasses to drizzle

Put the oats in a saucepan and cover with the water. Bring to the boil and gently simmer for a few minutes until the porridge thickens. Before serving, add the cashew nuts and linseed oil and stir in well. Serve drizzled with runny honey or molasses and pour over soya milk or whole milk as desired.

parsley eggs

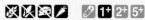

8 eggs
A splash of soya milk (or whole milk if dairy-tolerant)
A handful of chopped parsley
1 tbsp extra virgin olive oil (or a knob of butter if dairy-tolerant)

Beat the eggs together with the milk. Stir in the chopped parsley. In a frying pan, heat the oil or melt the butter. Add the egg and gently cook, stirring all the time until the egg thickens and is cooked through. Serve on wholemeal toast or with rye crackers, and a drink of fresh orange juice.
The orange juice will aid iron absorption from the egg.

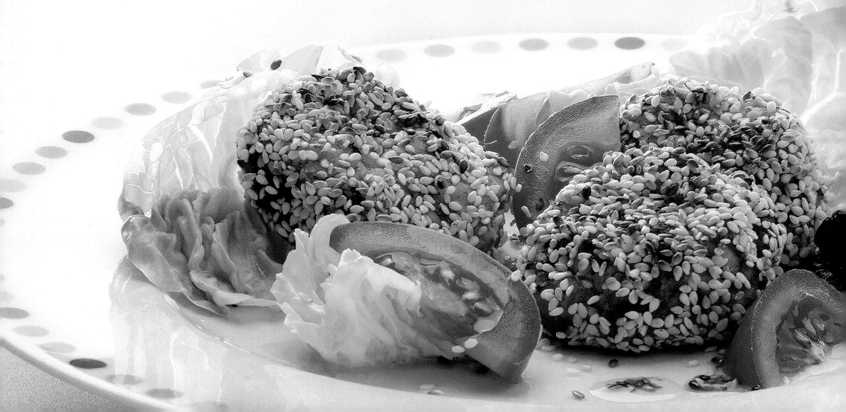

MAIN MEALS

turkey and cranberry burgers *below left*

1 onion, finely chopped
1 tbsp extra virgin olive oil
225 g (8 oz) minced turkey
1 eating apple, grated
2 tbsp cranberry sauce
2 medium potatoes, cooked and mashed
Sesame seeds for coating

Gently cook the onion in the olive oil until translucent. Add the turkey mince and cook, stirring constantly for 10 minutes or until it is cooked through. Take the mixture off the heat and mix in the rest of the ingredients except the sesame seeds. Allow to cool and then form small burgers with your hands. Place in the fridge for 30 minutes to set. Brush with olive oil and coat in sesame seeds. Grill for five minutes, turning frequently to stop the sesame seeds from burning. If your toddler doesn't like the sesame seed coating, you could coat them in the more traditional egg and breadcrumbs.

tuna fishcakes

1 fresh tuna steak
2 medium potatoes, peeled and chopped
1 medium onion, finely chopped
1 tbsp extra virgin olive oil
1 egg, beaten
A small handful of parsley, chopped
A splash of tamari soy sauce

Bake or steam the tuna steak for 20 minutes until cooked through. Cook and lightly mash the potatoes. Sauté the onion in a little olive oil until soft. Mix all of the ingredients together in a bowl and form into eight small fishcakes. Place in the fridge for 1 hour before cooking. Gently fry in a little olive oil until crisp on both sides.

toddler fish pie

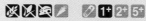

1 skinless and boneless cod fillet
1 salmon fillet
Enough soya milk (or whole milk if dairy-tolerant) to cover the fish
4 medium potatoes
1 tbsp unhydrogenated vegetable margarine (or a knob of butter if dairy-tolerant)
1 heaped tbsp gluten-free flour (or plain flour if wheat- and gluten-tolerant)
2 hard boiled eggs, chopped
A handful of fresh parsley

Preheat the oven to 180°C/350°F/Gas Mark 4. Place the cod and salmon in a pan on the hob and cover with the milk. Gently simmer for 15–20 minutes until the fish is cooked through. Remove the fish from the milk and place it in an ovenproof serving dish, reserving the milk in a measuring jug. Mash the fish up to make sure there are no bones. Meanwhile, boil the potatoes until cooked and then mash for the pie topping. In another saucepan, melt the margarine or butter. Add the flour and mix well. Slowly add the reserved milk to this pan, stirring constantly to prevent lumps. If lumps do form, use a hand whisk to eliminate them. When the sauce has thickened, remove from the heat and pour over the fish. Add the chopped eggs and parsley and mix well. Cover with the mashed potato and place in the oven for 30 minutes until the potato is crispy on top and the pie is hot throughout.

pheasant paysanne

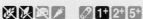

Game is rich in the immune-boosting minerals iron and zinc. This pheasant casserole can be enjoyed by any age group from toddlers upwards.

1 tbsp extra virgin olive oil
1 prepared pheasant
2 garlic cloves, crushed
1 onion, chopped
2 apples, peeled, cored and sliced
1 cup (225 ml/8 fl oz) cider or apple juice
2 tbsp natural yoghurt
A handful of chopped parsley

Preheat the oven to 180°C/350°F/Gas Mark 4. Heat the oil in a heavy-bottomed casserole dish. Add the whole pheasant and brown well. Remove the pheasant and place to one side. Add the garlic and onion to the pan and cook gently until the onion becomes translucent. Add the apple slices and cider and place the pheasant back in the pan. Baste the pheasant well, cover and place in the oven for 1½ hours. Once cooked, carve the pheasant and liquidize the sauce along with the natural yoghurt. Pour over the pheasant, sprinkle with the parsley, and serve with mashed potatoes and a green vegetable.

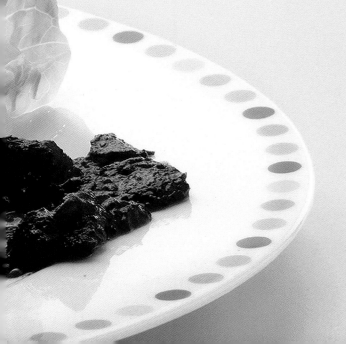

carrot and cashew nut soup

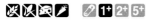 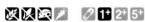

1 tbsp extra virgin olive oil
1 onion, chopped
A 500 g (1 lb 2 oz) bag of carrots, peeled and chopped
1 tsp ground coriander
850 ml (1½ pints) vegetable stock
1 small bag of cashew nuts, chopped
A small handful of fresh, chopped coriander plus a little extra to serve

In a saucepan, heat the olive oil and gently cook the onion until translucent. Add the carrots and ground coriander and stir well. Cover with the stock and simmer for 30 minutes until the carrots are soft. Add the cashew nuts and allow to cool. Add the fresh coriander and liquidize to form a thick soup. Sprinkle with chopped coriander and serve with croutons made from pieces of wholemeal toast or rice cakes.

sticky fingers chicken

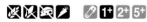

You may need to take the meat off the wings for very young toddlers.

MARINADE
2 garlic cloves, crushed
1 cm (½ inch) root ginger, grated
2 tbsp runny honey
Juice of 1 lemon
Grated rind of ½ a lemon
2 tbsp tamari soy sauce

12 chicken wings

Preheat the oven to 190°C/375°F/Gas Mark 5. Mix all of the marinade ingredients together in a glass jug. Put the chicken wings in a roasting pan and cover with the marinade. Leave to marinate for 30 minutes, turning the chicken halfway through. Bake in the oven for 35–40 minutes, basting after 15 minutes. The chicken will be very sticky to handle when cooked.

quick and easy beany bake

Another great teatime dish.

2–3 medium potatoes, peeled and chopped
1 small onion, finely chopped
1 tbsp extra virgin olive oil
1 tin of baked beans (no-sugar, no-salt variety)
1 tin of sweetcorn (no-sugar, no-salt variety)

First put the potatoes on to boil and preheat the oven to 190°C/375°F/Gas Mark 5. Meanwhile, in a saucepan, gently cook the onion in the olive oil until translucent. Add the baked beans and sweetcorn and heat through. Transfer to an ovenproof dish. When the potatoes are cooked, mash them with a little non-hydrogenated vegetable margarine (or butter if dairy-tolerant) and then cover the bean mixture with them. Place in the oven for 15–20 minutes until the potato has lightly browned.

homemade chicken fingers and chips

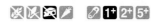

CHICKEN FINGERS
2 skinless and boneless chicken breast fillets
A handful of flour
2 eggs, beaten
2 pieces medium wholemeal bread made into breadcrumbs
A little olive oil for frying

CHIPS
1 potato per child
Extra virgin olive oil for brushing
Dried oregano

Preheat the oven to 190°C/375°F/Gas Mark 5. Chop the potatoes in half lengthways and then into quarters. Continue doing this until you have some chunky chip shapes. Put the shapes into a roasting tin, brush with olive oil and sprinkle with oregano. Cook for 40 minutes to 1 hour depending on the number of chips you are cooking. While the chips are cooking, slice the chicken breasts lengthways into long fingers. Coat them in the flour, roll them in the egg and then coat them in the breadcrumbs. In a frying pan, heat a little olive oil and gently fry the chicken fingers for about 15 minutes, turning several times.

make your own pizza *right*

 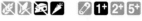

All children will love helping with this recipe.

1 cup (115 g/4 oz) wholemeal flour
1 cup (115 g/4 oz) plain flour
1 tsp mixed herbs
1 cup (225 ml/8 fl oz) lukewarm water
4 tbsp olive oil
1 sachet of instant yeast
A variety of toppings
2–3 tbsp tomato purée

Sieve the flour into a mixing bowl and mix in the herbs. Make a well in the middle of the flour. Pour in the water and the oil and add the yeast. Slowly mix the flour in with the liquid to form a stiff dough. If the dough is too dry, add a little more warm water. When the dough has formed, turn it out onto a floured surface and knead for a few minutes. Then put it back into the bowl and leave to one side while you prepare the toppings. On a large plate, set out a selection of toppings for the children to choose from, such as sliced onion, sliced peppers, grated carrot, grated beetroot, grated cheese, sliced mushrooms, tinned tuna chunks, pepperoni slices, cooked broccoli florets, cooked salmon, olives, basil leaves and anything else they might like. The combinations really are endless. Once prepared, divide the dough in two and roll out thinly into two circles. Spread the tomato purée on the top and decorate with the toppings. Bake in a hot oven (230°C/450°F/Gas Mark 8) for 20–25 minutes until the pizzas are crispy and the cheese is sizzling.

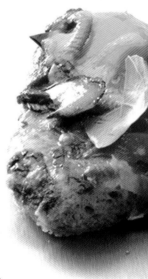

family salad

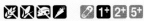

Children will love to help you prepare this salad and it is a great introduction to raw foods full of antioxidants and phytonutrients.

1 crunchy lettuce, washed and chopped
A handful of sprouted beans and seeds
1 carrot, peeled and grated
2 sticks celery, chopped
A few cherry tomatoes, sliced in half
½ cucumber, diced
A few toasted pumpkin and sunflower seeds
A handful of raisins
1 red pepper, diced

Place the washed lettuce in a large salad bowl and pile all the other ingredients on top. Serve with your child's favourite dressing (try Garlic and Honey Dressing, page 117).

sweetcorn patties

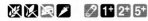

This makes an excellent teatime dish served with a crunchy salad.

1 tbsp chopped coriander
2 eggs, beaten
5 tbsp natural yoghurt
½ cup (60 g/2 oz) easy-cook polenta
1 tin of sweetcorn
2–3 tbsp extra virgin olive oil

Mix all of the ingredients except the oil together in a bowl. Heat the oil in a frying pan and drop spoonfuls of the mixture into the pan. Cook for roughly 5 minutes, turning the patties halfway through to make sure they are golden brown on both sides.

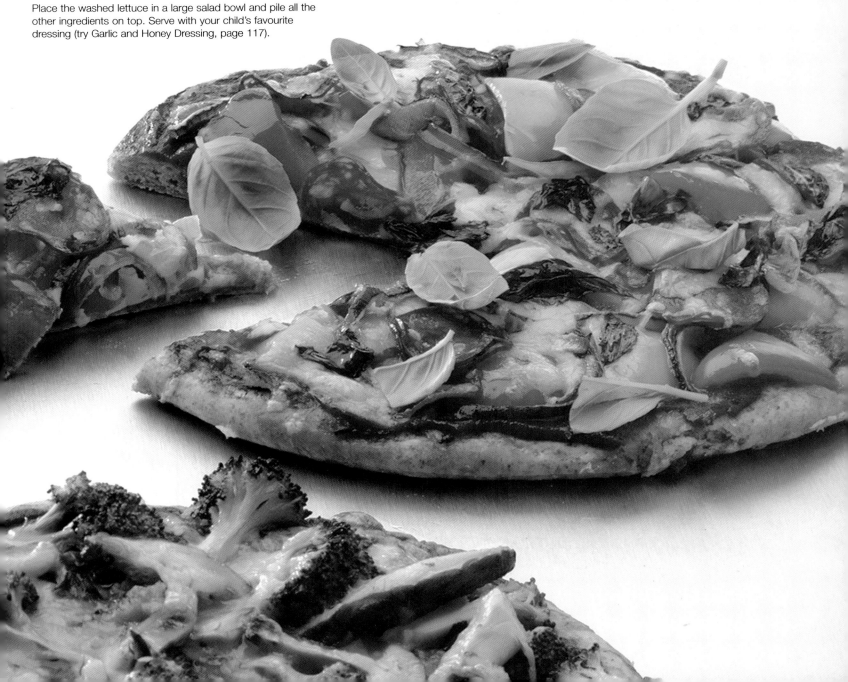

farmhouse lentil pie

 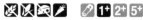

This is a wonderful vegetarian alternative to shepherd's pie. It is a good source of iron and a host of immune-boosting phytonutrients, and can be enjoyed by vegetarians and meat-eaters alike.

½ cup (100 g/3½ oz) green lentils
4 medium potatoes for mashing
A knob of vegetable margarine (or butter if dairy-tolerant)
1 large onion, chopped
1 garlic clove, crushed
1 tbsp extra virgin olive oil
A handful of shiitake mushrooms (stalks removed), chopped
1 tin of chopped tomatoes (no-sugar, no-salt variety)
1 tbsp tomato purée
1 tbsp tamari soy sauce
A handful of curly parsley, finely chopped

Put the lentils in a saucepan and cover them with water. Bring to the boil and gently simmer for 45 minutes until soft. Make sure they do not dry out – add more water as they cook if necessary. Drain them in a sieve and put to one side. Meanwhile, peel, chop and boil the potatoes until soft. Mash with a little vegetable margarine or butter and leave to one side. In another saucepan, lightly cook the onion and garlic in the olive oil until soft. Add the mushrooms and cook for a further couple of minutes. Add the cooked lentils, tomatoes, tomato purée and the soy sauce. Cook for a further couple of minutes and then take the pan off the heat. Add the chopped parsley, mix thoroughly and pour the mixture into an ovenproof dish. Cover with the mashed potato, using a fork to make lines over the top of the pie. Bake in a moderate oven (190°C/375°F/Gas Mark 5) for 30 minutes to heat through and lightly brown the mashed potato. Serve with a green vegetable or crunchy green salad and sugar-free tomato ketchup.

PUDDINGS AND BAKING

homemade yoghurt with help yourself toppings

 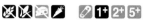

600 ml (1 pint) whole milk
1 heaped tsp live natural yoghurt

In a glass measuring jug, combine 1 tablespoon of the milk with the yoghurt. In a saucepan gently heat the rest of the milk until it is hot but not boiling. Pour the hot milk into the measuring jug and mix well. Pour the mixture into a vacuum flask and put the lid on. Leave to set in a warm place. This will take about 6 hours. Once set, transfer the yoghurt into a bowl or jug and store, covered, in the fridge for up to 5 days.

HELP YOURSELF TOPPINGS
In ramekins or muffin trays, set out a selection of toppings such as raisins, chopped banana, fresh strawberries, sliced kiwi fruit, blueberries, chopped up dried fruit bars, chopped sesame bars, runny honey, wheatgerm and grated chocolate. Spoon some yoghurt into a bowl and add some toppings!

design a bug

  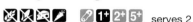   serves 2

1 orange, halved
A selection of chopped fruits
Raisins
Cocktail sticks

On a plate, place the orange flat side down. Arm yourself with the cocktail sticks and start designing your bug! Raisins are good for eyes and spots. Pineapple squares can be good for feet or arms. The mind boggles but your children will have great fun and will enjoy the fruit as well.

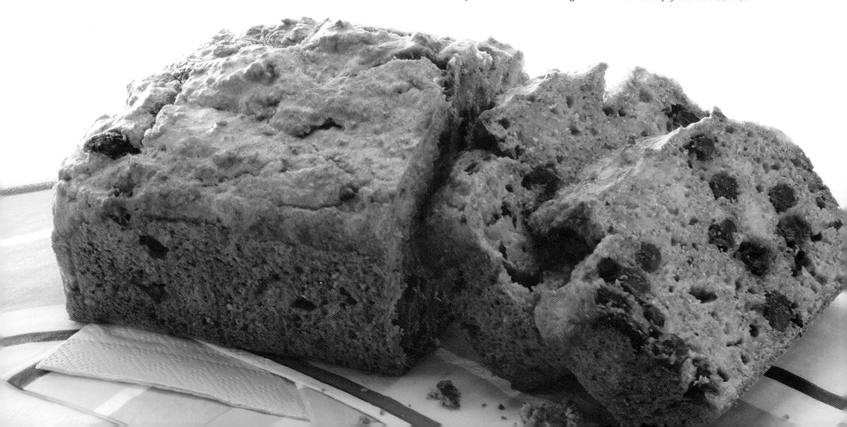

muesli squares

  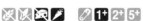   makes aproximately 28 squares

½ cup (75 g/2½ oz) chopped dried apricots
¼ cup (60 g/2 oz) fructose
½ cup (60 g/2 oz) mixed nuts, chopped
1 cup (100 g/3½ oz) oats
½ cup (75 g/2½ oz) raisins
¼ cup (30 g/1 oz) sesame seeds
½ cup (60 g/2 oz) wholemeal self-raising flour
2 tbsp runny honey
2 eggs, beaten
²/₃ cup (150 g/5½ oz) softened butter

Preheat the oven to 180°C/350°F/Gas Mark 4. Mix all of the dry ingredients together in a bowl. In another bowl, mix the honey, eggs and butter. Combine the ingredients. Transfer to a lightly-oiled shallow baking tin and bake for 20 minutes until golden brown.

banana and raisin cake *below left*

2 eggs, beaten
4 ripe bananas, mashed
1 tsp mixed spice
¹/₂ cup (75 g/2³/₄ oz) sun-dried raisins
¹/₃ cup (75 g/2³/₄ oz) softened unhydrogenated vegetable margarine (or butter if dairy-tolerant)
1 cup (115 g/4 oz) wholemeal self-raising flour

Preheat oven to 180°C/350°F/Gas Mark 4. Mix together the beaten eggs and the mashed bananas. Add the rest of the ingredients and stir well. Transfer to an oiled loaf tin and bake for 40 minutes until cooked through.

mango hedgehog

   1 mango (makes 2 hedgehogs)

Slice a mango down each side of the central stone. Score noughts and crosses through the flesh and then turn the mango slices inside out to create 2 mango hedgehogs.

dairy-free ice cream

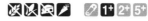

2 ripe bananas
½ cup (60 g/2 oz) cashew nuts, finely ground
1 tbsp maple syrup
1 tsp soya lethicin granules
1 cup (225 ml/8 fl oz) calcium-fortified soya milk

Blend all of the ingredients together in a liquidizer. Pour into a shallow freezer container and freeze for a couple of hours, mixing up with a fork after 1 hour. Remove from the freezer 10 minutes before serving.

DRINKS

strawberry smoothie

  Makes 2 large glasses or 4 small ones

1 cup (225 ml/8 fl oz) apple juice
2 ripe bananas
1 tbsp linseed (flaxseed) oil
1 small punnet of strawberries, destalked

Liquidize all the ingredients together and serve immediately.

kiwi and banana smoothie

Makes 2 large glasses or 4 small ones

1 cup (225 ml/8 fl oz) apple juice
2 ripe bananas
3 kiwi fruit, peeled
1 tsp linseed (flaxseed) oil
A pinch of vitamin C powder

Liquidize all the ingredients together and serve immediately.

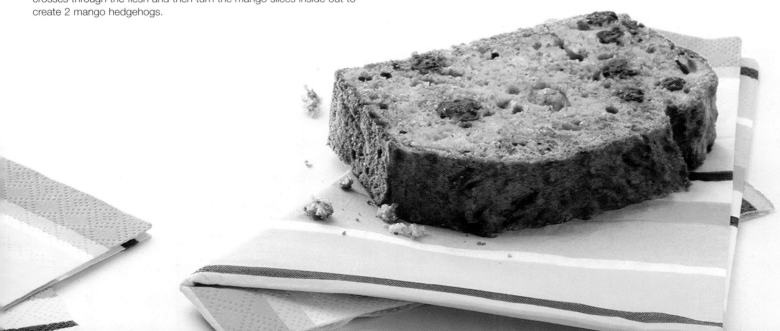

5–12 years

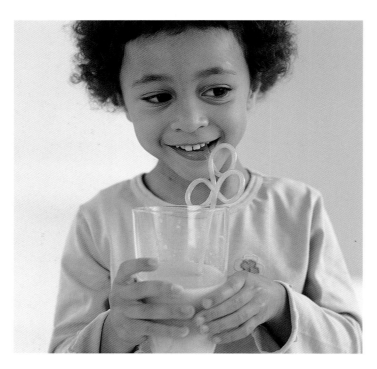

The school child's immune system

At around the age of five, your child will be ready to start school and this can be a very demanding time for his immune system. Although it has now developed enough to be operating efficiently and to create antibodies to any viruses it encounters, it will also come under greater pressure due to stress, a key immune system enemy. At school, there will be new and challenging pressures to face, such as learning to read and write, making friends and obeying new rules. These challenges, combined with exposure to a plethora of different bacteria and viruses, can put a strain on your child's immune system. If, however, you concentrate on supporting your child's immunity through a healthy diet, you will keep him vital and well equipped to cope with his new and exciting experiences.

Nutritional needs of school children

Your child's eating habits will be fairly well established by now. His healthy, balanced diet should include plenty of B-vitamins to cope with the demands of the school day. The B-vitamins are sometimes called the "stress vitamins" because they trigger the production of calming and mood-enhancing hormones. They also help to boost antibody activity and phagocytic activity (the process by which white blood cells engulf invading micro-organisms) and can be found in poultry, game, wholegrains, nuts, seeds and green leafy vegetables.

With the arrival of school and new friends, children in this age group will be regularly exposed to the temptations of junk food. Be sure to give them plenty of the antioxidants found in colourful fruits and vegetables as these help to protect against the free-radical damage that such foods can cause. Free radicals are rogue atoms that attack cells in the body, causing disease. Some are produced by the body's normal metabolic processes or by an immune system assault on a virus. Sometimes, however, too many are produced. Excessive free-radical production has been linked to factors such as environmental pollution and the eating of deep-fried or burnt foods, such as chips, chicken nuggets, barbecued meat or burnt toast. Antioxidants help mop up free radicals and we all need the extra ammunition provided by eating antioxidant-rich foods. Foods high in antioxidants are those that contain any of the vitamins A, C and E and the minerals selenium, copper and zinc. In addition, many of the phytonutrients found in fresh fruits and vegetables have antioxidant properties. In particular, beta-carotene, which is both a phytonutrient and the plant form of vitamin A, is a potent antioxidant and can be obtained from eating lots of brightly-coloured fruits and vegetables.

The school day is a long one, so it is imperative that you feed your child a diet that will help to sustain his energy throughout it. Being tired leads to lowered immunity. This may be the first time that your child will be having a meal away from home, either as a packed lunch or a school lunch. Most school food is of poor quality both in terms of taste and nutritional value so, if school lunch is compulsory, focus on breakfast and supper as the nutrient-rich meals of the day.

Your school-age child should be eating three meals a day and two to three snacks. Breakfast should combine both protein and complex carbohydrates. Protein helps to keep children alert by

SUGGESTED WEEKLY MENU PLANNER

	Monday	Tuesday	Wednesday	Thursday	Friday	Saturday	Sunday
breakfast	Crunchy Muesli (page 86) with sliced banana	Dry-fried Eggy Bread (page 86), orange slices	Creamy Cashew Porridge (page 78), pear slices	Nut Butter Sandwiches (page 86), fruit slices	Parsley Eggs (page 78) on toast, orange juice	Wholegrain cereal, Papaya and Lime Smoothie (page 91)	Fruity Scotch Pancakes (page 78), strawberries
snack			S E E	B O X	B E L O W		
lunch	Packed lunch or school lunch	Packed lunch or school lunch	Packed lunch or school lunch	Packed lunch or school lunch	Packed lunch or school lunch	Seafood Paella (page 66) with salad, Blackcurrant Ice Cream (page 90)	Roast chicken and vegetables, baked apple and custard
snack			S E E	B O X	B E L O W		
supper	Venison Sausages with Pea, Mint and Potato Mash (page 88), fruit, Banana and Raisin Cake (page 83)	Cod and Parma Ham Parcels with Red Pesto (page 89), fruit, 100% Fruit Jam Tarts (page 90)	Chicken and Almond Satay with Carrot and Sesame Stir-Fry (page 88), Crunchy Yoghurt Pudding (page 90)	Salmon Lollipops (page 89) with new potatoes and green beans, Pineapple and Mango Jelly (page 91)	The Very Best Vegetarian Burgers (page 86) with salad, Peach and Apricot crumble (page 90) with ice cream	Make Your Own Pizza (page 80), fruit, Muesli Squares (page 83)	Picnic or sandwich tea
snack			S E E	B O X	B E L O W		

lowering levels of the sleepy hormone serotonin, and complex carbohydrates release energy slowly, helping to keep blood sugar levels balanced during the morning. In practice, this could mean offering a boiled egg and wholemeal toast, homemade muesli and nut butter sandwiches or toast, fruity scotch pancakes, smoothies, or, when speed is essential, muesli bars with some fruit.

When children come back from school, have some good snacks ready. They need to eat more than three times a day to keep their energy up while they are growing. See the chart, right, for some ideas. Always have fruit in bowls around the house that they can help themselves to as and when they feel like it. Fruit provides plenty of important antioxidants and beneficial phytonutrients.

Supper should be a family affair whenever possible. It should contain lots of complex carbohydrates to balance blood sugar levels and help children unwind after a long day. Avoid sugary snacks in the evening, as they will not only suppress your child's immune system but they are also likely to excite rather than calm him before bedtime.

GOOD SNACK IDEAS

Fruit smoothie made with silken tofu or natural yoghurt

Fruit and fruit bars

Rice cakes with nut butter

Nut Butter Sandwiches (page 86)

Hummus with corn crackers

Banana and Raisin Cake (page 83)

Unsweetened popcorn

Apple and cheese sticks

Smoked mackerel pâté on toast

Nut and seed bars

Muesli Squares (page 83)

Mixed nuts and raisins

Corn on the cob with almond butter

5–12 years recipes

These recipes are designed for two adults and two children unless otherwise stated in the recipe itself. All ingredients, where possible, should be organic to protect young immune systems.

BREAKFASTS

Here are some more energy-packed breakfast ideas for school children. The breakfast recipes listed for the other age groups would also be good for this age group.

crunchy muesli *right*

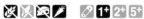

This recipe keeps for 2 weeks in an air-tight container and can be doubled or tripled depending on how quickly it gets eaten.

¼ cup (30 g/1 oz) linseeds (flaxseeds)
2 tbsp maple syrup
½ cup (60 g/2 oz) mixed nuts, chopped
¼ cup (30 g/1 oz) pumpkin seeds, chopped
1 cup (100 g/3½ oz) rolled oats
¼ cup (30 g/1 oz) sunflower seeds, chopped
2 tbsp walnut oil

Preheat the oven to 180°C/350°F/Gas Mark 4. Place all the ingredients into a mixing bowl and combine well. Turn out into a shallow baking tin and bake in the oven for about 20 minutes until golden brown and well toasted. You will need to stir the muesli once or twice during the cooking time. Leave to cool and then store in an airtight container. Serve with milk, soya milk, yoghurt or fruit juice, topped with some chopped banana.

dry-fried eggy bread

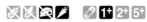

An instant hit with all age groups.

8 eggs, beaten
A splash of soya milk (or whole milk if dairy-tolerant)
4 thick slices wholemeal bread

Beat the eggs with the milk. Pour the mixture onto a serving plate. Lay out the bread on top and leave to soak for a few minutes. Turn the bread over and wait until the bread has absorbed most of the egg. Heat a non-stick frying pan and when really hot add the egg-soaked bread. Gently dry-fry the bread until golden brown and the egg is cooked through. You can cut out shapes for children with pastry cutters or serve whole.

nut butter sandwiches

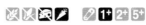

These sandwiches provide plenty of energy as well as calcium, iron, fibre and essential fats for your child.

1 cup (115 g/4 oz) chopped nuts (choose which type your child likes best: almonds or cashews, walnuts or peanuts)
A couple of tbsps of raisins
A little olive oil or walnut oil
2 slices wholemeal bread per child

Blend the nuts and raisins together in a food processor to make a thick paste. This will take some time. Add a little oil to get the right consistency and to help the blending process. Spread one slice of the bread with some of the nut butter. Put the other slice on top to make a sandwich and cut into four. You can store any leftover nut butter in an airtight jar in the fridge for up to 2 weeks.

MAIN MEALS

the very best vegetarian burgers

    makes 16 small burgers

These burgers can be made in bulk and frozen on baking sheets lined with greaseproof paper. Once frozen, transfer to freezer bags and keep for up to 1 month.

175 g (6 oz) green lentils
1 small carrot, finely grated
1 stick celery, finely grated
1 tsp Dijon mustard
1 egg, beaten
2 garlic cloves, crushed
2 tsp mixed herbs
1 packet (125 g/4 oz) mixed nuts, ground in food processor
1 small onion, finely chopped
3 medium slices wholemeal bread made into breadcrumbs
A splash of Worcestershire sauce
Sesame seeds for coating

Pre-cook the lentils by simmering them in a pan filled with water for 45 minutes until soft. Drain well. Put all of the ingredients together in a mixing bowl and mix well. Form into 16 burgers and coat with the sesame seeds. Place on a baking sheet, brush with olive oil and grill for 6–8 minutes each side. Serve with salad, coleslaw and sugar-free tomato ketchup.

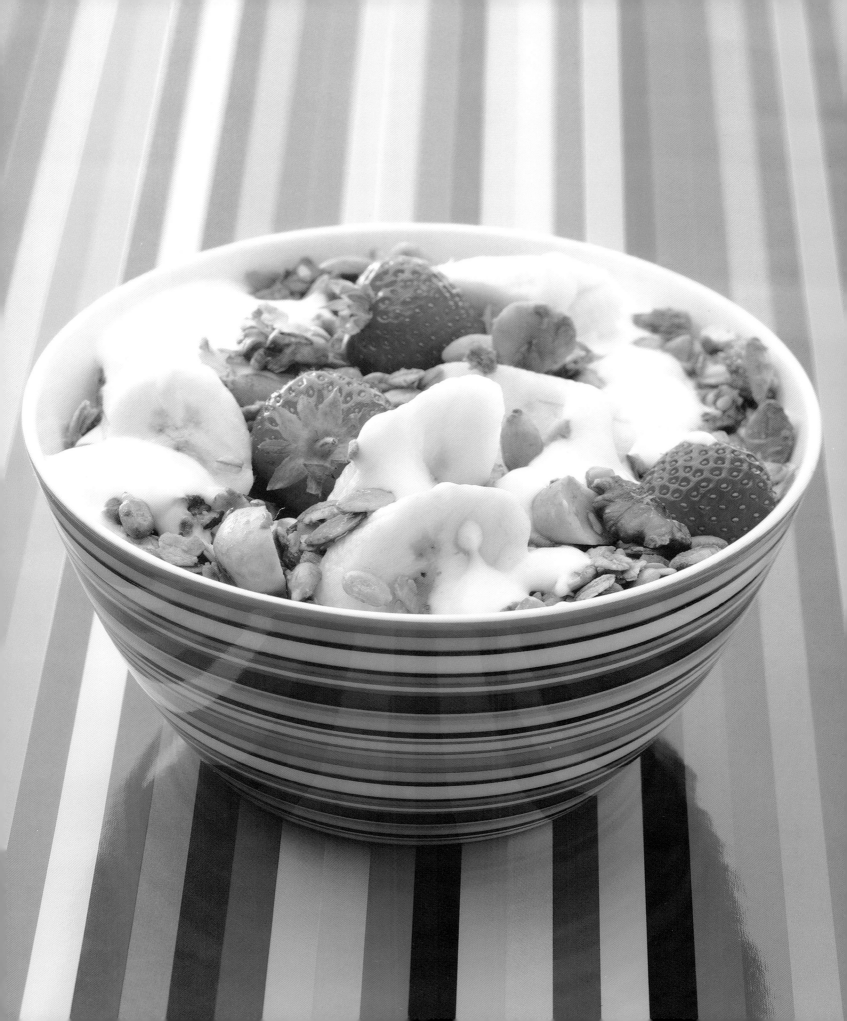

venison burgers

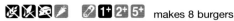 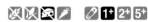 makes 8 burgers

Venison is low in fat and an excellent source of iron and zinc.

1 tbsp date syrup
1 egg, beaten
1 large onion, finely chopped
1 tsp dried thyme
250 g (9 oz) minced venison
1 tbsp extra virgin olive oil

Combine all the ingredients except the oil in a mixing bowl. Form round, flat, mini-burger shapes about an inch thick. Heat the olive oil in a frying pan. When really hot, add the burgers and cook for 3–4 minutes each side. Serve in wholemeal pittas packed out with shredded salad and dressing.

venison sausages with pea, mint and potato mash

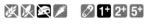

12 venison sausages
4 medium potatoes, peeled and quartered
1 cup (150 g/5½ oz) fresh peas
A few mint leaves

Grill the venison sausages until cooked through. Meanwhile, boil the potatoes with the mint leaves for 15–20 minutes. Add the peas and cook for another 5 minutes. Drain the vegetables, remove the mint and mash the potatoes and peas together with a little unhydrogenated margarine or butter. Sprinkle a little finely chopped mint on the top of the potatoes to serve.

finger lickin' chicken with BBQ sauce

6–8 chicken drumsticks
Olive oil for brushing
A little dried oregano

BBQ SAUCE:
1 garlic clove, crushed
1 small onion, finely chopped
1 tbsp extra virgin olive oil
1 tbsp apple cider vinegar
1 tsp Dijon mustard
2 tbsp runny honey
½ tsp molasses
2 tbsp Worcestershire sauce

Brush the chicken drumsticks with olive oil and sprinkle with a little oregano. Place them under the grill and cook for 10–12 minutes each side, depending on the size, until cooked through. Meanwhile, in a saucepan, gently cook the garlic and the onion in the olive oil until soft. Add the rest of the ingredients and simmer gently for 5 minutes. Serve alongside the chicken drumsticks with a large crunchy salad.

chicken and almond satay with carrot and sesame stir-fry *below*

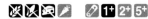

2 chicken breasts
3 tbsp almond butter (this is available from all good supermarkets and health-food shops)
2 tbsp tamari soy sauce
2 tbsp water
8 wooden satay sticks or barbecue sticks, soaked in water for 30 minutes to prevent burning

Cut each chicken breast into four strips. Combine the almond butter, tamari soy sauce and water in a dish, coat the chicken strips with this mixture and then thread them onto the satay sticks. Arrange the sticks on a lightly oiled baking tray and cook under a grill for 12–15 minutes, turning a couple of times, until the chicken is cooked through and the outside is golden brown.

CARROT AND SESAME STIR-FRY
1 bundle of rice noodles
1 tbsp extra virgin olive oil
4 carrots, peeled and cut into batons
A handful of sesame seeds
A splash of tamari soy sauce

In a heat-proof bowl, soak the rice noodles in boiling water for 5 minutes. Heat the oil in a wok. Add the carrots and stir-fry for 3–4 minutes. Toss in the sesame seeds and the soy sauce and stir-fry for a further couple of minutes. Drain the rice noodles and add to the stir-fry pan. Serve in Chinese bowls topped with the chicken satay.

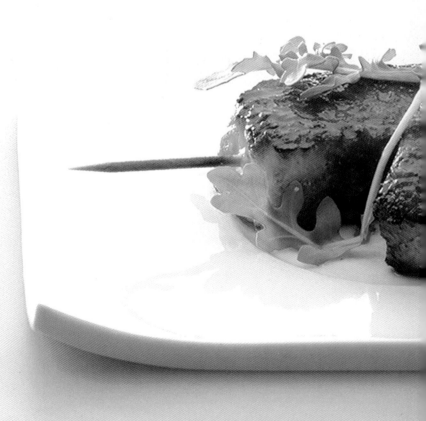

tuna and prawn brochette
with coriander marinade

 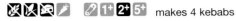 makes 4 kebabs

8 cherry tomatoes, whole
2 small courgettes, cut into 8 chunks
8 peeled tiger prawns
1 tuna steak, cut into 8 chunks
4 kebab sticks, soaked in water for 30 minutes to prevent burning

MARINADE
A small handful of fresh coriander
1 garlic clove, crushed
1 tbsp runny honey
1 tbsp lemon juice
2 tbsp tamari soy sauce

Mix all of the marinade ingredients together in a bowl. Push the fish and vegetables alternately onto the kebab sticks and lay in a shallow baking dish. Lightly brush the kebabs with the marinade. Pour any remaining marinade into the dish and leave to soak for 30 minutes, turning occasionally so that the kebabs are well covered. Grill for 4 minutes each side until cooked through. Serve with steamed broccoli and brown rice.

cod and parma ham parcels with red pesto

 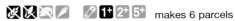 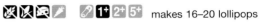 makes 6 parcels

2 skinless and boneless chunky cod loins
6 strips Parma ham
Red pesto, for spreading

Preheat the oven to 190°C/375°F/Gas Mark 5. Cut each piece of fish into three. On an oiled baking tray, lay out a strip of the Parma ham. Lightly spread the Parma ham with the red pesto. Place the cod fillet in the middle. Fold up the sides over the fish and then fold over the ends to cover the fish. Turn the parcel over to neaten the edges. Do this with all six of the fish portions and lay them out on the baking tray. Bake for 15–20 minutes until the fish is cooked through. Serve with green beans and new potatoes.

salmon lollipops

  makes 16–20 lollipops

2 large and chunky salmon fillets, skinned
3 tbsp mild curry powder
3 tbsp runny honey
1 tbsp extra virgin olive oil
16–20 cocktail sticks, soaked in water for 30 minutes to prevent burning

Cut each salmon fillet into 8–10 pieces. On a plate, mix the curry powder and honey together to make a paste. Mix in the oil. Roll the salmon pieces in the sauce and place on the cocktail sticks. Put the lollipops on an oiled baking sheet and cook under a hot grill for 10 minutes, turning halfway through.

egg and veggie bake

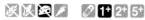 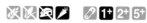

5 eggs, beaten
½ cup (115 g/4 oz) extra virgin olive oil
1 cup (115 g/4 oz) plain flour
1 tsp baking powder
3 courgettes, grated
1 large onion, chopped
1 tin of sweetcorn
A handful of diced pancetta or streaky bacon
1 cup (115 g/4 oz) grated cheese (optional)
A splash of soya milk (or whole milk if dairy-tolerant)

Preheat the oven to 180°C/350°F/Gas Mark 4. Lightly oil an ovenproof dish. In a large bowl, mix the eggs, oil, flour and baking powder together. Add the courgette, onion, sweetcorn, pancetta and cheese and add some milk if the mixture is too stiff. Pour the mixture into the dish and bake for 30–40 minutes until browned.

PUDDINGS AND BAKING

popcorn

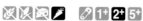

2 tbsp extra virgin olive oil
Enough popcorn to cover the bottom of a stainless steel pan

Heat the oil in the pan and add the popcorn. Place a lid on the pan and, shaking it from time to time, wait until the popcorn starts popping. Keep the pan on a gentle heat until the popping subsides and continue to shake it now and again to prevent the popcorn from burning.

crunchy yoghurt pudding with summer fruits compote

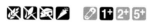

600 ml (1 pint) homemade yoghurt (see page 51)
A few homemade digestive biscuits (see right)

SUMMER FRUITS COMPOTE
A punnet of each of the following: strawberries, blackberries, blueberries and raspberries
3 tbsp filtered water
1 heaped tbsp fructose

Preheat the oven to 190°C/375°F/Gas Mark 5. Prepare the berries and chop any large strawberries into smaller pieces. Place all of the fruit in an ovenproof dish with the water, sprinkle over the fructose and cover the dish with foil. Bake in the oven for half an hour until the fruit is soft and there is a good amount of juice at the bottom. Allow to cool. Put the yoghurt in a serving bowl and fold in the compote. Crumble the biscuits over the yoghurt and refrigerate to chill before serving.

peach and apricot crumble

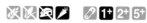

10 ripe apricots, peeled, stoned and halved
5 ripe peaches, peeled, stoned and chopped
½ tsp nutmeg
2 tbsp runny honey
¼ cup (60 g/2 oz) orange juice

CRUMBLE TOPPING
½ cup (60 g/2 oz) ground almonds
2 tbsp fructose
⅓ cup (75 g/2¾ oz) unhydrogenated vegetable margarine (or softened butter if dairy-tolerant)
½ cup (60 g/2 oz) wholemeal flour

Preheat the oven to 190°C/375°F/Gas Mark 5. Prepare the fruit and place in a lightly-oiled ovenproof dish. Sprinkle with the nutmeg, drizzle over the honey and pour the orange juice around the fruit. Meanwhile, place the crumble ingredients into a blender and blend very lightly until they resemble breadcrumbs. Do not over-blend or you will be left with a dough. Mix the crumble with your hands if you prefer. Cover the fruit with the crumble and bake in the oven for 30 minutes until the topping is golden brown.

blackcurrant ice cream *right*

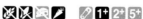

1 tin of blackcurrants in juice
¼ cup (60 g/2 oz) fructose
1 600 ml (1 pint) pot of natural yoghurt

Gently heat the blackcurrants and their juice with the fructose until the sugar has all dissolved. In a mixing bowl, combine the yoghurt with the blackcurrant mixture and allow to cool. Once cooled, transfer to a plastic freezer box and freeze until set. This should take a couple of hours. You will need to bring the ice cream out of the freezer every half an hour and stir it round to make it set well and prevent it from becoming a solid frozen block.

100% fruit jam tarts

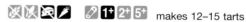 makes 12–15 tarts

1 cup (115 g/4 oz) wholemeal flour
1 tsp baking powder
2 tsp walnut oil or linseed (flaxseed) oil
¼ cup (60 g/2 oz) unhydrogenated vegetable margarine (or butter if dairy-tolerant)
3 tbsp water
100% fruit jam (no added sugar)

Preheat the oven to 180°C/350°F/Gas Mark 4. For the pastry cases, combine the flour and baking powder in a mixing bowl. Add the rest of the ingredients except the jam and mix to form a dough. Wrap the dough in clingfilm for half an hour. Then remove the clingfilm and roll out the dough very thinly. Using a pastry cutter, cut out small rounds to fit a jam-tart baking tray. Lightly oil the moulds, place a pastry round in each one and add a teaspoon of fruit jam. Bake for 20 minutes until the pastry is cooked. Allow to cool and serve.

pineapple and mango jelly

1 mango, diced
600 ml (1 pint) natural pineapple juice
2 sachets of vegegel or other vegetarian alternative

Place the chopped mango into a jelly mould. Put the pineapple juice into a saucepan and add the vegegel. Gently heat to boiling point, stirring all the time to ensure that the vegegel dissolves. Pour over the mango, allow to cool slightly, and place in the fridge for a few hours until it sets.

homemade digestive biscuits

     makes 20 biscuits

1 cup (115 g/4 oz) self-raising wholemeal flour
1 cup (175 g/6 oz) fine oatmeal
A pinch of sea salt
1 tsp baking powder
½ cup (115 g/4 oz) unhydrogenated vegetable margarine (or softened butter if dairy-tolerant)
¼ cup (60 g/2 oz) fructose
4 tbsp soya milk (or semi-skimmed milk if dairy-tolerant)
1 tbsp sesame seeds

Preheat the oven to 190°C/375°F/Gas Mark 5. Mix the flour, oatmeal, salt and baking powder together in a bowl. Rub in the margarine until the mixture resembles breadcrumbs. Mix in the fructose. Add the milk to form a dough. Roll out thinly on a lightly-floured surface. Cut out the biscuits with pastry cutters, prick them and brush with water. Sprinkle with sesame seeds, place on an oiled baking sheet and bake for 10 minutes.

DRINKS

These smoothies are a wonderful way of serving fruit. One small cup will supply your child with their daily requirement of antioxidant vitamins. They can be made quickly to accompany breakfast, or as a snack. Without the added juice they can be served as a fruit fool pudding. Alternatively, try freezing the smoothie in lolly moulds to make a summertime treat.

papaya and lime smoothie

    makes 2 large glasses or 4 small ones

2 bananas
Juice of 1 lime
1 tbsp linseed (flaxseed) oil
1 cup (225 ml/8 fl oz) orange juice
1 papaya

Whizz all the ingredients up in a liquidizer and serve immediately.

cranberry and apple smoothie

    makes 2 large glasses or 4 small ones

2 apples, cored and chopped
1 cup (225 ml/8 fl oz) apple juice
1 banana
1 small punnet of cranberries
1 tbsp linseed (flaxseed) oil

Whizz up all the ingredients in a liquidizer and serve immediately.

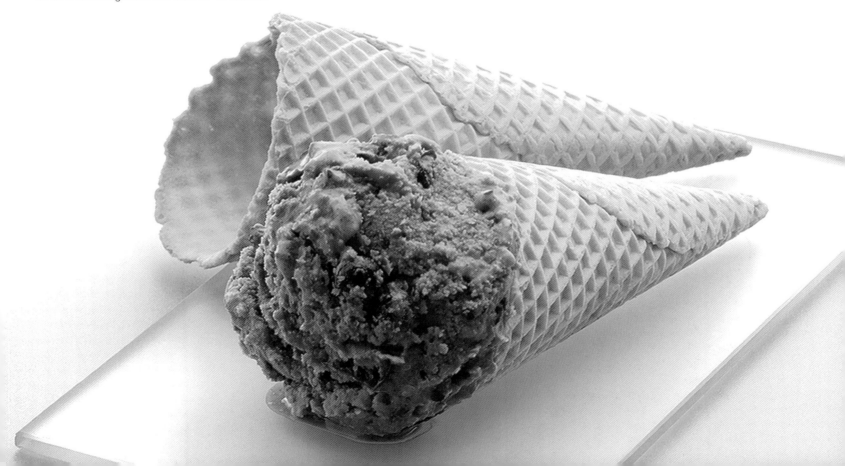

13–18 years

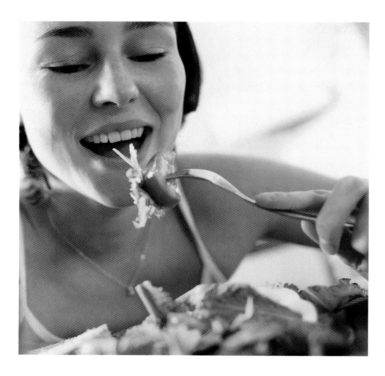

Nutritional needs of teenagers

The teenage diet needs to support the body through the changes caused by puberty and, in particular, needs to address the rise of sex hormones occuring at this time, as these can have an adverse effect on the immune system. For girls, the beginning of menstruation and increases in their levels of oestrogen mean that they require a significant supply of iron. This important mineral enables red blood cells to carry oxygen around the body and supplies are often found to be low in teenage girls. This has a knock-on effect on their immune systems, making them more susceptible to infection. Good sources of iron are dried fruit, green leafy vegetables, poultry, game, red meat, lentils and egg. The rise in oestrogen also affects how they utilize magnesium and vitamin B6 and they will need increased levels of both. Low levels of magnesium affect antibody production and essential fatty acid metabolism, worsen PMS and increase allergic reactions. Foods rich in magnesium are nuts, seeds, green leafy vegetables, egg yolks, wholegrains and dried fruits.

Boys going through puberty need increased levels of zinc, which is concentrated in their semen. The only way to replace the zinc is through their diet. Zinc is an immune-boosting antioxidant which is also important for reproductive and skin health. Low levels will result in more frequent colds and infections. Good sources of zinc are poultry, game, shellfish, nuts, seeds and wholegrains.

All teenagers need a good all-round supply of antioxidant vitamins and minerals to help protect them from pollution and increase resistance to disease. Foods high in antioxidants are those that contain any of the vitamins A, C and E and the minerals selenium, copper and zinc. Vitamin E is especially important for teenagers as it helps to maintain healthy skin, which is often a problem for this age group. You should also try to ensure that your teenager receives plenty of B-vitamins as these, too, are good for skin health as well as for maintaining energy levels and growth, and stimulating the production of the anti-stress hormones serotonin and dopamine. Foods rich in B-vitamins include nuts and seeds, poultry, game, wholegrains and green leafy vegetables.

Immune boosting for teenagers

Once your child hits the teenage years, his immune system will be well developed. However, it is not without reason that these are often called the "turbulent years", and your teenager will be going through many changes. Not only will his body be changing, but he will also face the pressure of important exams and the stress that often accompanies them. Stress can have a profound effect on the immune system. Children can get stressed about things not perceived as stressful to adults, and immune deficiency can occur from repeated exposure to the stressors that they find threatening. Common stressors are worries about school work, bullying, recurrent infections (such as tonsillitis) or an unhappy home life. Raised levels of the stress hormone cortisol will cause immune suppression, resulting in reduced levels of antibodies and lowered resistance to infection. While it is obviously key to support your teenager's emotional needs at this time, a good diet will help arm bodies and minds with the nutrients required to keep them in optimum health.

SUGGESTED WEEKLY MENU PLANNER							
	Monday	Tuesday	Wednesday	Thursday	Friday	Saturday	Sunday
breakfast	Crunchy Muesli (page 86) with sliced banana	Breakfast in a Glass (page 94)	Tropical Fruit Salad with Seeds and Live Yoghurt (page 94)	Yoghurt Crunch with Summer Fruits Compote (page 94)	Boiled egg with toast	Strawberry Smoothie (page 83)	Toast with nut butter
snack			S E E	B O X	B E L O W		
lunch	Packed lunch or school lunch	Packed lunch or school lunch	Packed lunch or school lunch	Packed lunch or school lunch	Packed lunch or school lunch	Rustic Saturday Soup (page 95) with wholemeal bread	Roast chicken with vegetables, baked apple and custard
snack			S E E	B O X	B E L O W		
supper	Sweet and Sour Prawn Stir-Fry with Egg Noodles and Bok Choi (page 96)	Spaghetti with Fresh Tomato, Avocado and Pine Nut Pasta Sauce with Balsamic Vinegar (page 97)	Fish Parcels (page 96) with rice and steamed vegetables	Chicken with Butternut Squash and Coconut (page 96) with rice and broccoli	Vegetable Frittata (page 96) with salad	Gazpacho (page 94), Stir-fry Duck Strips with Orange and Ginger (page 97) with noodles	Pasta with Nutty Pesto (page 39) with salad
snack			S E E	B O X	B E L O W		

The teenage daily diet should consist of three meals and two or three snacks. Healthy snacks between meals are still important for this age group as they keep blood sugar levels stable, thus helping to maintain levels of concentration throughout the school day. The aim is to combat the reliance that many teenagers have on fast food and unhealthy snacks as their main food supply, and to address the accompanying peaks and troughs in their energy and concentration. In particular, they should avoid fizzy drinks as much as possible as these are full of phosphorous, artificial colours and flavours, sugar, sweeteners and preservatives. The high phosphorous levels leach important minerals, including calcium, zinc and magnesium, from your child's body. Make fizzy drinks an occasional option in your house and not one that is available all of the time. Breakfast can be unpopular, especially with teenage girls, so preparing a liquid meal may be the answer. A quick shake or smoothie as they rush out of the door can contain all the nutrients required to sustain them through the morning. Lunch will either be a packed lunch or a school lunch and supper usually eaten at home.

GOOD SNACK IDEAS

Fruit, and fruit smoothies and shakes

Mixed nuts and raisins

Fruit, nut and seed bars

Muesli Squares (page 83)

Sesame and Honey Bars (page 99)

Hummus with carrot and celery sticks or toast

Rice cakes with cashew butter

Banana and Raisin Cake (page 83)

Unsweetened popcorn

Cheese and apple

Ryvita (crispbreads) with smoked mackerel dip

Oatcakes with nut butters or cottage cheese

Crudités, grissini sticks and dips

Tropical Fruit Salad with Seeds and Live Yoghurt (page 94)

13–18 years recipes

These recipes will serve four adults unless otherwise stated in the recipe itself. All ingredients should be organic, where possible.

BREAKFASTS

breakfast in a glass *right*

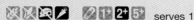   serves 1

This is a great way of serving up a nutritious breakfast to even the most reluctant teenager. This sumptuous liquid meal will keep them going right through their morning's studies.

1 cup (225 ml/8 fl oz) apple juice
1 ripe banana
A handful of seasonal berries
1 tbsp linseed (flaxseed) oil
1 tbsp pumpkin seeds
1 tsp natural wheatgerm
1 cup (350 g/12 oz) plain soya yoghurt (or homemade yoghurt if dairy-tolerant)

Blend all the ingredients together in a liquidizer to make a delicious and filling smoothie.

tropical fruit salad with seeds and live yoghurt

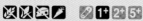 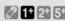

Especially popular with girls, this fruit salad has a little of all that is needed to set your teenager up for the day.

½ cantaloupe melon, cut into chunks
2 kiwi fruit, peeled and chopped
1 mango, peeled and cut into chunks
1 papaya, deseeded and cut into chunks
¼ watermelon, cut into chunks
1 cup (225 ml/8 fl oz) fresh orange juice
Soya yoghurt (or live yoghurt if dairy-tolerant), to serve
Toasted seeds to sprinkle

Prepare all the fruit and combine in a serving dish with the orange juice. Serve in bowls topped with yoghurt and sprinkled with lightly toasted seeds.

yoghurt crunch with summer fruits compote

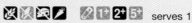   serves 1

This is just as delicious topped with sliced banana instead of the Summer Fruits Compote.

½ cup (100 g/3½ oz) Crunchy Muesli (page 86)
2 tbsp soya yoghurt (or live yoghurt if dairy-tolerant)
1 tbsp Summer Fruits Compote (page 90)

Place the muesli in a bowl or glass. Top with yoghurt and add a spoon of Summer Fruits Compote.

MAIN MEALS

gazpacho

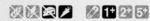

Another wonderfully easy recipe that can sit and wait in the fridge for a late teenager! Served with crunchy French bread and some cheese, it makes a meal in itself at any time of day or night.

1 onion, chopped
2 slices medium cut white bread, crusts removed
2 red peppers, deseeded
½ cucumber, peeled
1 garlic clove, crushed
4 celery sticks
2 cups (450 ml/16 fl oz) tomato passata
1 cup (225 ml/8 fl oz) water
3 tbsp extra virgin olive oil
3 drops Tabasco sauce
A generous pinch of sea salt
Freshly ground black pepper
Diced onion, red pepper and cucumber for serving

In a food processor, whizz up the onion to a fine pulp. Add the bread, red peppers, cucumber, garlic and celery. Blend together until finely chopped. Add the passata, water, olive oil and Tabasco. Blend the mixture together until smooth. Season the soup to taste and refrigerate until needed. Finely chop some red peppers, onion and cucumber to add to the gazpacho when serving.

rustic saturday soup

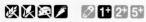

This is one of my favourite winter Saturday lunches for the family. Served with hunks of wholemeal bread, it makes a filling, earthy meal full of immune-boosting nutrients.

1 onion, chopped
A handful of chopped pancetta or streaky bacon
1 garlic clove, crushed
2 tbsp extra virgin olive oil
2 carrots, peeled and chopped
2 sticks celery, chopped
A pinch of cayenne pepper (optional)
2 tins of chopped tomatoes
1 tin of chickpeas (no-sugar, no-salt variety)
1 cup (225 ml/8 fl oz) vegetable stock

In a saucepan, gently cook the onion, pancetta and garlic in the olive oil for a few minutes. Add the carrots and celery and stir well. Sprinkle over the cayenne pepper and mix it around with the vegetables. Add the chopped tomatoes, chickpeas and vegetable stock and simmer for 20 minutes until the vegetables are soft.

homemade soda bread

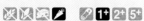

250 g (9 oz) wholemeal flour
250 g (9 oz) plain flour
2 tsp bicarbonate of soda
A knob of unhydrogenated margarine (or butter if dairy-tolerant)
1 heaped cup of homemade yoghurt

Preheat the oven to 190°C/375°F/Gas Mark 5. In a mixing bowl, combine the flour and bicarbonate of soda. Add the butter and yoghurt to form a dough. Mould the dough into a round loaf and place on a baking tray. With a knife, mark a cross on the top and bake in the oven until the loaf has risen and is golden brown and crusty on top. Remove from the oven and leave to cool on a wire rack. Serve immediately. If kept, soda bread is best eaten toasted.

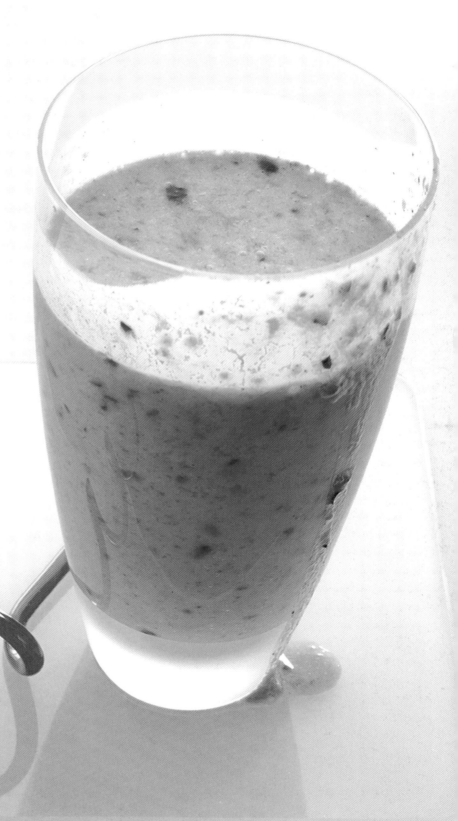

smoked mackerel dip

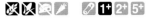

This takes minutes to prepare and is delicious as a dip with crudités and grissini sticks. It also serves as a starter with Homemade Soda Bread (page 95).

1 tbsp horseradish sauce
2 smoked mackerel fillets, skinned
1 handful of flat leaf parsley
1 small pot (125 g/4 oz) live natural yoghurt or homemade yoghurt

In a food processor, whizz all the ingredients together to make a smooth paste. Refrigerate before serving.

fish parcels

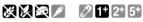

1 bunch of fresh coriander
3 garlic cloves, crushed
1 dice-sized piece ginger, thinly sliced
Juice of 2 limes
1 small bunch of spring onions
4 chunky fish fillets (such as seabass or cod)
8 rice paper circles (available from oriental supermarkets)

Preheat the oven to 190°C/375°F/Gas Mark 5. In a food processor, mix together all of the ingredients except the fish and the rice papers until finely chopped. Tip into a mixing bowl. Coat each of the fish steaks with the mixture and place on a plate. Dip the rice paper circles in hot water to soften them. Lay them out on a plate and place the fish steaks in the middle. Wrap each fish fillet in 2 rice papers and brush with oil. Place on a baking sheet and cook for 20–25 minutes until the fish is cooked through. Serve with stir-fried vegetables and rice.

chicken with butternut squash and coconut

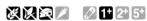

1 red onion, chopped
1 garlic clove
2 tbsp extra virgin olive oil
1 chicken, cut into 8 portions (ask your butcher to prepare it)
1 butternut squash, peeled and chopped
1 tin of coconut milk
2 medium potatoes
600 ml (1 pint) vegetable stock
Some freshly chopped coriander and parsley to serve

Preheat the oven to 190°C/375°F/Gas Mark 5. In a heavy bottomed casserole pan, gently cook the onion and garlic in the oil until translucent. Add the chicken pieces and cook to seal on both sides, turning occasionally. Add all of the rest of the ingredients except the herbs, bring to the boil and cover. Place in the oven and cook for one hour until the chicken is cooked. Once cooked, skim off any excess fat. Sprinkle with chopped coriander and parsley and serve with brown rice and your choice of a green vegetable.

vegetable frittata

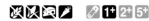

3 spring onions, finely chopped
1 medium potato, diced small
2 tbsp extra virgin olive oil
1 carrot, grated
1 courgette, grated
2 tbsp peas
8 eggs
A splash of soya milk (or semi-skimmed milk if dairy-tolerant)
1 tbsp fresh coriander, chopped

In a deep frying pan, gently cook the onions and diced potato in the olive oil until the onions are soft and the potato browned. Add the rest of the vegetables and allow them to cook for a couple of minutes. Beat the eggs together with the milk and the herbs and pour over the vegetables. Shake the frying pan to ensure that the egg covers all the vegetables. Turn the heat really low and gently cook until the underside is nicely browned. Loosen the omelette and take off the heat. Using oven gloves, place a large, flat baking sheet on top of the frying pan and flip the omelette onto it. Then slide the omelette back into the pan and continue cooking until the underside is brown and the omelette cooked through. Serve in wedges with a crunchy salad.

sweet and sour prawn stir-fry with egg noodles and bok choi

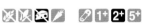

This is popular with all children over the age of two.

2 portions nest egg noodles
3 tbsp extra virgin olive oil
1 garlic clove, crushed
1 dice-sized piece ginger, grated
300 g (10 oz) raw, peeled tiger prawns
¼ cup (60 ml/2 fl oz) pineapple juice
1 tbsp tomato purée
1 tbsp cider or white wine vinegar
A pinch of paprika powder
1 packet of bok choi, sliced
A splash of tamari soy sauce
1 tsp runny honey

Boil the egg noodles according to the instructions on the packet. Heat a couple of tablespoons of the oil in a wok. Add the garlic and ginger. Cook for about a minute and then add the prawns. Stir-fry for 3–4 minutes until the prawns have turned pink. Add the pineapple juice, tomato purée, vinegar and paprika powder and cook for a further couple of minutes until the sauce thickens and the prawns are cooked through. Drain the noodles and add them to the stir-fry pan. Toss them through and take the wok off the heat. Place the contents of the wok in a hot serving dish and cover while you cook the bok choi. Wash the wok and put a tablespoon of oil in the bottom. Heat the wok, add the bok choi and stir-fry for a couple of minutes. Add a splash of tamari soy sauce and the honey. Toss the bok choi in the soy sauce for a further minute and serve immediately with the prawns and noodles.

fresh tomato, avocado and pine nut pasta sauce with balsamic vinegar *below*

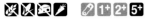

4 large ripe tomatoes
2 garlic cloves, crushed
1 avocado, diced
A handful of pine nuts, toasted under the grill
A handful of basil leaves, shredded
2 tbsp balsamic vinegar
Enough corn spaghetti (or wholewheat spaghetti if gluten-tolerant)
    for 4 people

Soak the tomatoes in boiling water for a couple of minutes to loosen their skins. Skin the tomatoes, remove the hard core and chop them into a serving bowl. Add the crushed garlic, diced avocado, toasted pine nuts and basil to the bowl. Sprinkle the balsamic vinegar over the top and fold all of the ingredients together. Cook the spaghetti and drain well. Combine with the pasta sauce and serve immediately.

stir-fry duck strips with orange and ginger

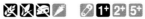

Juice of 1 orange
Zest of ½ an orange
1 tbsp runny honey
1 tbsp extra virgin olive oil
3 spring onions, sliced
1 garlic clove, peeled and crushed
2 thin slices root ginger
2 skinless duck breasts, cut into thin strips
12 baby sweetcorn

Mix the orange juice, orange zest and honey together in a bowl. In a wok, heat the oil and stir-fry the spring onions, garlic and ginger for a couple of minutes. Add the duck and stir-fry for another 2–3 minutes. Add the orange and honey sauce and the baby sweetcorn and stir-fry for a further 3–4 minutes until the sauce has reduced and the duck is cooked through. Serve with brown rice.

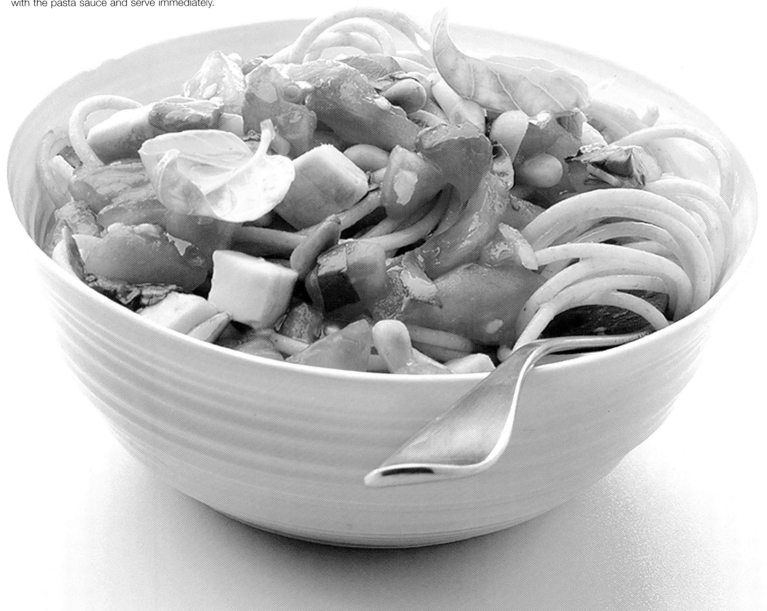

family paella

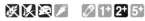

1 onion, chopped
2 garlic cloves, crushed
2 tbsp extra virgin olive oil
1 packet of diced pancetta
2 skinless and boneless chicken breasts
A pinch of turmeric
375 g (13 oz) brown rice or paella rice
850 ml (1½ pints) vegetable stock
1 green pepper, deseeded and diced
1 red pepper, deseeded and diced
1 cup (175 g/6 oz) frozen prawns (defrosted)
1 cup (175 g/6 oz) frozen peas
1 tin of sweetcorn (no-sugar, no-salt variety)
A handful of chopped flat leaf parsley

In a paella pan, gently cook the onion and garlic in the oil. Add the pancetta pieces, chicken and turmeric and cook until the meat has browned. Add the rice and coat with the oil. Add the stock and bring to the boil. Simmer, stirring frequently, for 25–30 minutes adding the peppers, prawns, peas and sweetcorn after 15 minutes' cooking time. Sprinkle with parsley and serve.

queen scallop stir-fry

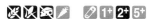

1 tbsp tamari soy sauce
1 tsp runny honey
1 tbsp white wine
1 tbsp extra virgin olive oil
1 red onion, thinly sliced
2 garlic cloves, crushed
1 tsp grated ginger
450 g (1 lb) queen scallops
1 small red pepper, deseeded and cut into strips
½ cup (75 g/2¾ oz) fresh peas
10 baby sweetcorn

In a bowl, mix the tamari soy sauce, honey and white wine together. Heat the oil in a wok and add the onion, garlic, ginger and scallops and stir-fry for 1–2 minutes. Add the pepper, peas and baby corn and stir-fry for 1 minute. Add the sauce and stir-fry for 3–4 minutes until the vegetables begin to soften and the scallops are cooked through. Serve with rice or noodles.

hot salad with balsamic dressing and fresh anchovies

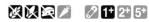

A large handful each of rocket leaves, watercress leaves
    and baby leaf spinach leaves
1 red onion, sliced
3 tbsp extra virgin olive oil
A punnet of new potatoes, cooked and halved
2 tbsp balsamic vinegar
8–10 fresh anchovy fillets

Place the salad leaves in a salad bowl. In a frying pan, gently cook the red onion in 1 tablespoon of olive oil. Add the cooked potatoes and continue cooking for a couple of minutes until the red onion begins to brown. Toss the potato mixture over the salad. Drizzle over the balsamic vinegar and add the remaining olive oil. Toss the salad together. Lay out the anchovy fillets on top of the salad in a star shape and serve immediately.

PUDDINGS AND BAKING

watermelon and ginger ice *below*

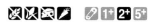

½ watermelon, cut into chunks
2 tbsp ginger cordial

In a liquidizer, whizz up the watermelon to a smooth purée. Pour into a shallow plastic tub and stir in the ginger cordial. Cover and place in the freezer for about 3 hours. Remove the mixture every 20 minutes for the first hour to stir and break up the ice particles.

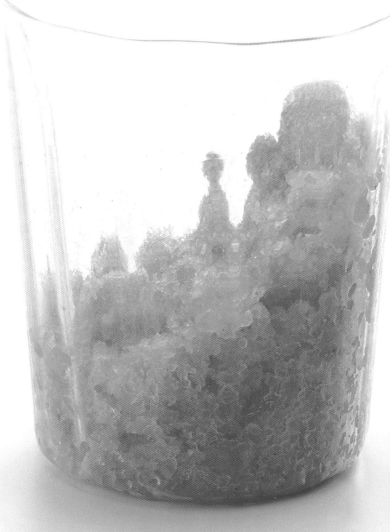

ginger and pear crumble

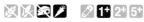

4 pears, peeled, decored and sliced
1 tsp grated root ginger

CRUMBLE TOPPING
¼ cup (75 g/2¼ oz) unhydrogenated vegetable margarine (or softened
    butter if dairy-tolerant)
½ cup (100 g/3½ oz) dark muscovado sugar
A handful of oats
1 tbsp sesame seeds
1 tbsp wheatgerm
½ cup (60 g/2 oz) wholemeal flour

Preheat the oven to 190°C/375°F/Gas Mark 5. Place the pears and the
ginger in an ovenproof dish. To make the crumble, put all the ingredients
into a mixing bowl and rub together with your fingertips until they resemble
fine breadcrumbs. Cover the fruit with the topping. Bake for 20–30 minutes
in the oven until topping is golden brown. Serve with a little soya cream or
natural yoghurt if desired.

summer pudding

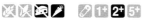

4–5 slices white or brown bread, crusts removed
Summer Fruits Compote (page 90)

Line a 1-pint pudding basin with most of the bread, cutting the pieces
so that they fit all the way around. Tip the Summer Fruits Compote into
the bowl and then cover with a layer of bread. Place a side plate on top
of the bowl and put something heavy on top of the plate. This adds some
weight to the mixture and helps the bread to soak up the juices. Allow the
pudding to soak overnight in the fridge. Before serving, turn out the
summer pudding onto a plate and cover with any extra juice remaining in
the bowl. Serve with homemade yoghurt or ice cream.

sesame and honey bars

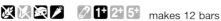   makes 12 bars

1 cup (100 g/3½ oz) sesame seeds
1 cup (175 g/6 oz) oatmeal
½ cup (175 g/6 oz) runny honey
½ cup (115 g/4 oz) unhydrogenated vegetable margarine (or butter if
    dairy-tolerant)
A pinch of sea salt

Preheat the oven to 180°C/350°F/Gas Mark 4. In a food processor, roughly
grind the sesame seeds and the oatmeal together. In a saucepan, melt the
honey and margarine, add the salt and then pour the mixture into the food
processor. Blend and turn out into a well-oiled baking tray about 25 cm/10
ins square. Bake for 25–30 minutes, or until golden brown. It is easiest to
cut the biscuits in the tin and then leave them to cool before removing.

healthy apple strudel

   makes 16 parcels

1 bag (450 g/1 lb) eating apples, peeled, cored and halved
½ cup (75 g/2¼ oz) sun-dried raisins
¼ cup (30 g/1 oz) flaked almonds
2 tsp ground cinnamon
1 tsp grated lemon rind
2 tsp maple syrup
2 pieces medium-cut wholemeal bread made into breadcrumbs
1 packet of filo pastry squares
A little melted unhydrogenated vegetable margarine (or butter if
    dairy-tolerant)

Thinly slice the apples and place in a mixing bowl along with the raisins,
almonds, cinnamon, lemon rind and maple syrup. Add the breadcrumbs
and mix well. Lay out the filo pastry squares on a baking sheet, brush with
a little melted margarine. Add 1–2 tablespoons of the apple mixture into
the middle of each square. Carefully fold up each parcel and brush with
margarine on the outside. Repeat until all the mixture has been used.
Bake for 25 minutes at 100°C/225°F/Gas Mark ¼ and then for a further
20 minutes at 180°C/350°F/Gas Mark 4. Serve with crème fraîche or
dairy-free ice cream.

DRINKS

nectarine and cherry smoothie

  makes 2 large glasses or 4 small ones

1 cup (225 ml/8 fl oz) apple juice
2 bananas
10 cherries, destoned
1 tbsp linseed (flaxseed) oil
2 nectarines, peeled and destoned

Whizz up all the ingredients in a blender and serve immediately.

melon, grape and banana smoothie

  makes 2 large glasses or 4 small ones

1 cup (225 ml/8 fl oz) apple juice
1 banana
½ cantaloupe melon
1 tbsp linseed (flaxseed) oil
2 tbsp natural yoghurt
A handful of seedless red grapes

Whizz up all the ingredients in a blender and serve immediately.

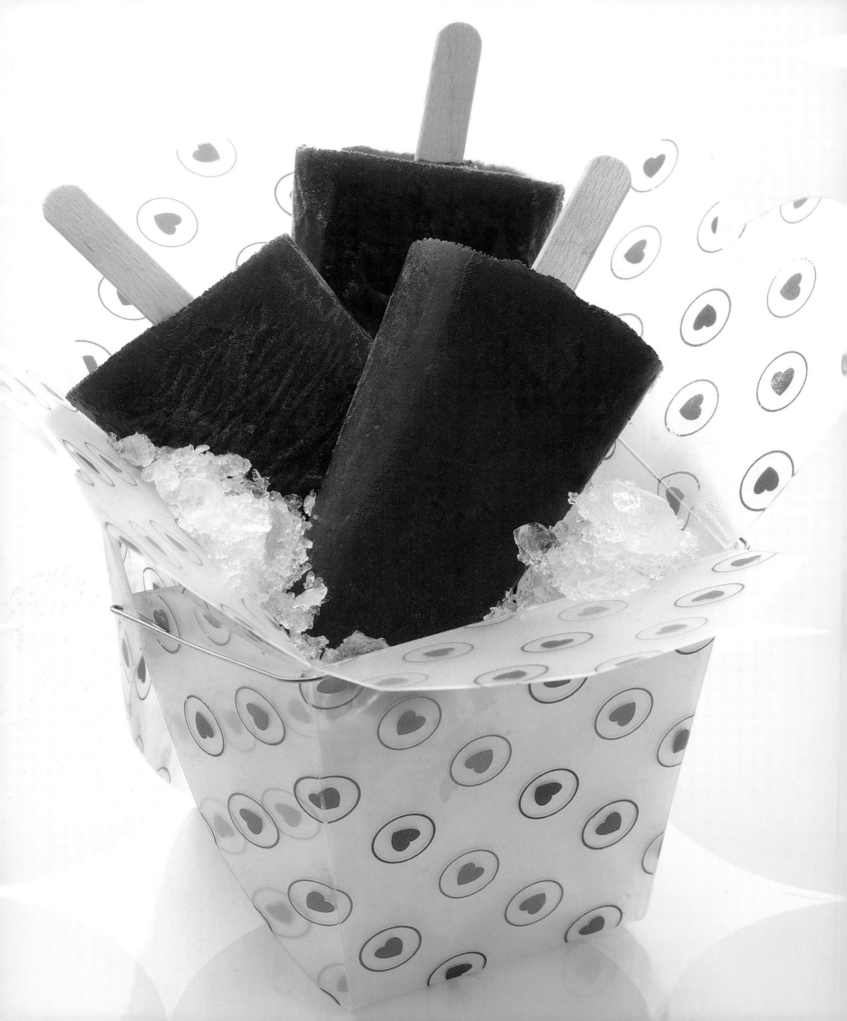

foods to fight common illnesses

However healthy your child's diet is, she will inevitably catch colds and other viruses from the environment in which she lives. Indeed, being exposed to the illnesses around her is an important part of her immune development. Part Four teaches you how to recognize and manage illnesses as they arise and how to use food to help in the healing process, providing detailed information on the most appropriate nutrients to include in your child's diet and where to find them. Advice on coping with each ailment is presented alongside restorative recipes designed to combat the unpleasant symptoms, comfort your child and give her immune defences a boost on the road to recovery. All recipes serve four unless otherwise stated.

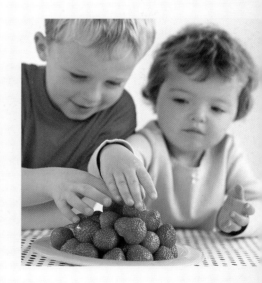

asthma

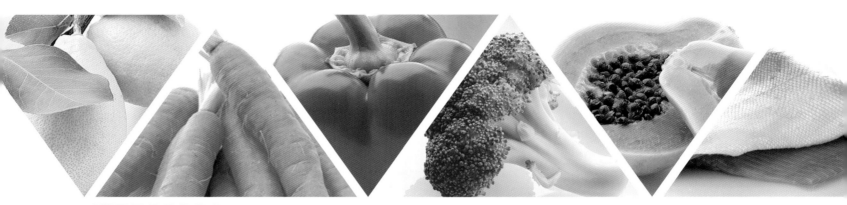

STAR FOODS FOR ASTHMA: ALMOND, BLACKCURRANT, BROCCOLI, BROWN RICE, CARROT, CHILLI, CINNAMON, CLOVE, FRESH TUNA, GARLIC, GINGER, HERRING, HORSERADISH, LEMON, LIME, MACKEREL, MANGO, MILLET, PAPAYA, PARSLEY, QUINOA, RED PEPPER, SALMON, SQUASH, SUNFLOWER SEED, THYME, WATERCRESS

Asthma is an inflammatory respiratory condition that causes difficulty in breathing. Symptoms can range from a dry cough, which is particularly bad at night, to a tight chest and heavy wheezing. It is caused by the constriction and swelling of the child's airways due to spasms in the bronchial tubes of the lungs. During an attack, there is also an increase in mucus secretions, which further inhibits the movement of air. An asthma attack can be fatal, so it is vital to seek medical advice if your child develops the condition.

Asthma tends to be more common in boys than girls and also where there is a familial history of allergic conditions such as hay fever or eczema. A child who has eczema as a baby has a higher risk of going on to develop asthma as a child. It is a disease that now affects one in five children in the UK, making it the country's most prevalent childhood illness (National Asthma Campaign). Worldwide, asthma in children has increased dramatically over the past 20 years. Various factors have been blamed for this increase, including environmental pollution and the fact that children in the developed world eat less fish, fruit and vegetables and consume more fatty foods than they did two decades ago. Also, our houses have become better insulated and can therefore retain certain known triggers of asthma, such as dust mites, moulds and pollen.

Every asthmatic child will have her own particular set of triggers that may precipitate an attack and these are important to identify and avoid. Common triggers are cigarette smoke, dust and dust mites, pets, pollen, exercise, exposure to cold weather, colds and viral infections, food additives, moulds, stress, laughter, some medicines such as aspirin, and cleaning products and perfumes.

Medicinal foods for asthma

Diet has an important role to play in the prevention and management of asthma. Many asthmatics have food allergies that can exacerbate their symptoms. Keeping a food diary can be a helpful way of establishing any food triggers. Common foods that can cause problems for asthmatic children include cow's milk, wheat, yeast, foods containing moulds (such as blue-veined cheeses), nuts, fish and egg. Certain food additives can also trigger an asthma attack in susceptible children so, if you have an asthmatic child, get to know your food labels. It is wise to avoid all benzoates (E210–219), sulphites (E220–228), gallates (E310–312) and yellow colourings (E102, E104 and E110). In addition, BHA (E320) and BHT (E321), which are added to certain oils and fats, should also be avoided.

A child with asthma should be on a wholefood diet full of fruits and vegetables, grains, lean proteins and without unnecessary saturated fat or sugar. They should eat plenty of foods rich in magnesium, a natural bronchodilator that can help to prevent spasms of the bronchial passages. Studies have shown that magnesium levels are often low in asthmatics. Good food sources of magnesium include nuts and seeds, green leafy vegetables, wholegrains and unsulphured dried fruit.

Incorporating plenty of oily fish into your child's diet also has a beneficial effect if she suffers from asthma. Mackerel, salmon, fresh tuna, sardines, herring and fresh anchovies are marvellous sources of omega-3 essential fatty acids, which suppress the formation of leukotrienes that can cause the bronchial tubes to constrict. If your child is asthmatic, prepare a meal of oily fish once a week to ensure she receives the omega-3 fats she needs.

Asthmatics tend to be low in B-vitamins and in vitamin C. These vitamins are not stored in the body, so need to be consumed on a daily basis. Foods rich in B-vitamins include wholegrains, pulses and green leafy vegetables and may help asthmatics, particularly those whose attacks are brought on by stress. Vitamin C is found in a wide range of fruits and vegetables, especially guava, kiwi fruit, citrus fruits, blackcurrants and peppers. Vitamin C is a powerful antioxidant, which means that it boosts your child's health generally by battling the harmful free radicals in the body that can cause disease and, more specifically in relation to asthma, it can help to strengthen the lungs and mucous membranes. Other foods rich in antioxidants are those containing vitamins A and E, and the minerals zinc, copper and selenium. Flavonoids, the phytonutrients (see page 140) found in many fruits and green vegetables, also have strong antioxidant properties. Make sure that your child eats five portions of fruit and vegetables a day to maintain a decent intake of antioxidants. A good rule of thumb is to remember that the more colourful the fruit or vegetable, the greater its antioxidant content.

Asthmatics should drink plenty of water and diluted fruit juices as these help to thin mucus secretions. Cooking with plenty of warming spices is also beneficial for the lungs. Such spices, which include ginger, chilli and cinnamon, have antiseptic and expectorant properties and can help relieve the symptoms of asthma.

SUGGESTED RECIPES FOR ASTHMA

ginger toddy
makes one mug

1 slice root ginger
Juice of 1 lime
1 cup (225 ml/8 fl oz) boiling water
1 tsp Manuka honey

Place the slice of ginger in the bottom of a mug. Squeeze in the lime juice and pour over the boiling water. Stir in the honey and allow the toddy to infuse for 5 minutes before drinking.

magnesium broth

1 tbsp extra virgin olive oil
2 garlic cloves, chopped
1 slice chilli (optional)
2 handfuls of green leafy vegetables, such as watercress, spinach, broccoli or rocket
1 cup (225 ml/8 fl oz) vegetable stock
2 tbsp ground almonds

In a saucepan, heat the oil and gently cook the garlic and chilli for a couple of minutes. Add the vegetables and stir until wilted. Pour in the vegetable stock, bring to the boil, cover and simmer for 15 minutes until the vegetables are cooked through. Liquidize the soup with the ground almonds and serve with wholemeal or rye toast.

salmon and broccoli risotto

1 onion, chopped
1 garlic clove, crushed
2 tbsp extra virgin olive oil
2 large boneless salmon fillets, cubed
1½ cups (300 g/10 oz) brown rice
1 litre (1¾ pints) vegetable stock
1 head of broccoli, broken into florets
A handful of fresh parsley

Gently cook the onion and garlic in the olive oil until translucent. Add the salmon and cook for a couple of minutes. Stir in the rice so that it is coated with the oil and then pour in about half of the vegetable stock. Bring to the boil and gently simmer for 25 minutes, adding more stock as needed. Add the broccoli and cook for a further 10 minutes or until the rice and broccoli are soft and the stock has been absorbed. Sprinkle with parsley to serve.

candida

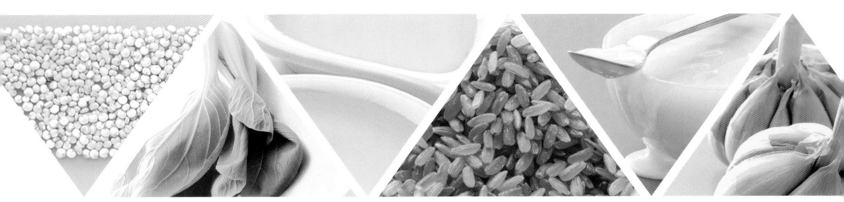

STAR FOODS FOR CANDIDA: BROWN RICE, CARROT, FRESH TUNA, GARLIC, GREEN BEANS, GREEN LEAFY VEGETABLES, HERRING, LEEK, LIVE YOGHURT, MACKEREL, MILLET, OLIVE OIL, ONION, QUINOA, SALMON, SARDINE, WHOLEMEAL FLOUR

The condition now commonly known as candida was first described as recently as 1978. Although many eminent doctors have published work on the condition, there remains today a great deal of controversy over candida, and many in the medical profession deny that it even exists. This is largely because there was an over-diagnosis of the problem in the 1980s at a time when candida became big business among alternative practitioners.

Candida Albicans is a yeast that inhabits the gut. It is a natural part of the plethora of good and bad bacteria inside the body that play an important role in general health. In a healthy child, the good bacteria will far outweigh the bad. These good bacteria are part of your child's first line of defence against harmful microbes. They produce B-vitamins, help to improve digestion and increase your child's resistance to gastrointestinal infection. They also produce substances that can act as natural antibiotics within the gut. Providing that there is equilibrium within your child's gut, the bacteria can all get along happily with each other. There are factors in the modern world, however, that place this equilibrium in jeopardy.

Today, children are exposed to antibiotics with increasing frequency and starting from a very young age. Antibiotics kill bacteria. They are not discriminatory and, as well as killing the bacteria causing the infection for which they were originally prescribed, broad-spectrum antibiotics will also kill the good bacteria in your child's gut. The routine use of antibiotics, combined with the high-sugar diet that most children consume, can result in an imbalance

in the gut and a weakened immune system. This encourages the bad bacteria to proliferate and to outweigh the good bacteria. If the yeasts in your child's gut grow out of control, they can turn into a pathogenic (disease-causing) form leading to increased permeability of your child's gut wall. The pathogenic form of the candida yeast also releases powerful toxins into your child's bloodstream, which can cause unpleasant symptoms such as tiredness, headaches, tummy aches, increased wind, bloatedness, food cravings, allergies, anxiety, skin rashes and poor concentration. These often accompany other fungal-type symptoms, such as thrush and athlete's foot.

If your child does show a combination of these symptoms it is advisable to ask your doctor or a qualified naturopath to test for a yeast overgrowth. There is some debate among health professionals about whether the yeast involved is in fact candida, but I have retained the common name for this condition for ease of reference. You might also hear it referred to simply as "yeast overgrowth".

The no yeast, no sugar diet

If your child has tested positive for a yeast overgrowth, diet plays the most important role in addressing the condition. A period of both yeast- and sugar-exclusion is the best way to restore the bacterial balance in the gut. Remember that when undertaking such a stringent diet to address a medical problem, especially if the sufferer is a child, you should always do so with the advice and guidance of a qualified healthcare professional.

The yeast in food is different from the yeast in your child's gut, but children with a yeast overgrowth become very sensitive to products containing yeast and such products should be eliminated from the diet for a period of a few months. Removing yeast from the diet involves avoiding all risen bread products, such as pizzas, croissants and breadsticks, yeast extracts including Marmite and Vegemite, all types of mushrooms, stock cubes, gravy powders, fermented foods such as soy sauce, miso and vinegar, and any packaged food with yeast on the label. Avoiding yeast can be very easy. There are now many ready-made yeast-free breads or you can make your own (see below). Yeasts feed off sugar, so it is very important to avoid all sugar while treating the problem, thus depriving the yeasts of their fuel. Eliminate all sweet foods, including cakes, pastries, puddings, biscuits, soft drinks, honey, dried fruit, jams and fruit concentrates. You can now find many good cookery books that deal with food avoidance.

Probiotics

Probiotics are live bacteria that can replenish your child's gut with the friendly bacteria it needs. They contain a balance of the bacteria commonly found in the human gut. Foods containing probiotics need to be refrigerated to survive and must be taken on a daily basis. A good food source is live yoghurt or live soya yoghurt. You can either make your own (see page 51) or buy it from supermarkets or health food shops. Probiotics are also available in a powdered form.

SUGGESTED RECIPES FOR CANDIDA

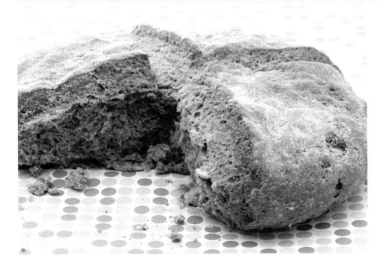

yeast-free bread

450 g (1 lb) wholemeal flour
A pinch of sea salt
2 tsp bicarbonate of soda
1 heaped cup (300 ml/10 fl oz) live yoghurt
A knob of butter, melted, or 1 tbsp extra virgin olive oil

Preheat the oven to 190°C/375°F/Gas Mark 5. In a mixing bowl combine the flour, the salt and the bicarbonate of soda and mix well. Make a well in the middle and pour in the yoghurt and melted butter or oil. If very thick, add a little water to thin slightly. Combine the ingredients to form a dough. Mould the dough into a round, flat-bottomed shape and place on a lightly-oiled baking tray. With a knife make a criss cross on the top and bake in the oven for about 30 minutes until it has risen and is golden brown and crusty on top. Remove from the oven and leave to cool on a wire rack. Soda bread tastes best when freshly baked. If kept, it is best toasted.

potato pizza

6 medium potatoes, peeled
A couple of sprigs of thyme, leaves removed and chopped
A pinch of salt and freshly ground black pepper
1 garlic clove, crushed
2 tbsp extra virgin olive oil
½ cup (115 ml/4 fl oz) tomato passata
A large handful of grated soya cheese (or mozzarella if dairy-tolerant)

Preheat the oven to 230°C/450°F/Gas Mark 8. Finely slice the potatoes on a mandolin or with the slicer on a food processor to get them really thin. In a mixing bowl, combine the potatoes, thyme, salt, pepper and garlic. Pour the oil into a non-stick frying pan and carefully layer the potato slices one on top of the other to create a circular potato base. Press the base down with a spatula so that it is well compacted. Gently cook the base over a medium heat until the bottom is lightly brown and crispy. Brush the top of the pizza base with some extra oil and transfer it to a lightly-oiled baking tray. Bake in the oven for 15–20 minutes until the potato is cooked through. Spread the passata over the potato pizza base and sprinkle the cheese over the top. Put back in the oven for a further 10 minutes until the cheese has melted. You can add a huge variety of other toppings – see page 80 for suggestions.

coughs

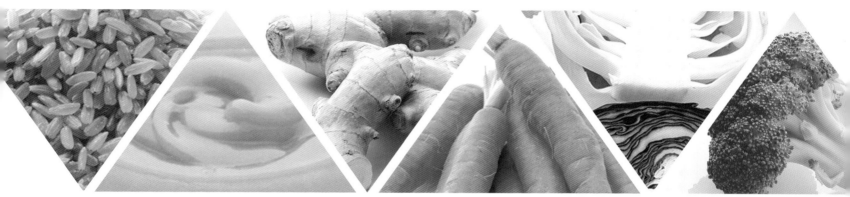

STAR FOODS FOR COUGHS: APRICOT, BROCCOLI, BROWN RICE, CABBAGE, CARROT, CINNAMON, COURGETTE, FENNEL, GARLIC, GINGER, HONEY, HORSERADISH, LEEK, LEMON, LETTUCE, LIME, MANGO, MANUKA HONEY, ONION, ORANGE, PAPAYA, PARSLEY, PUMPKIN, SWEET POTATO, THYME

Coughs are among the most common childhood ailments your child is likely to encounter. They are most prevalent in the winter months and often accompany colds, which help to prime and strengthen young immune systems. Coughing is an involuntary mechanism designed to clear your child's airways of dust, bacteria, viruses and other unwanted substances. A cough can be caused by viral or bacterial infections or by environmental allergens such as dust, pollen or cigarette smoke. Persistent coughs need medical attention, as they may be a symptom of a more serious disease. A cough that is accompanied by wheezing and difficulty breathing is most likely to be caused by asthma. A "barking" cough that sounds like a seal and is worse at night could be croup, an inflammation of the throat that can cause difficulty in breathing. A persistent cough that is accompanied by a fever and difficulty breathing could be caused by bronchitis, bronchiolitis or even pneumonia. If you suspect that your child may be suffering from any of these ailments, seek medical attention immediately.

If the cough is worse at night then it is important to elevate your child's head by propping her up with extra pillows. In the case of a baby, place a pillow or folded blanket underneath her mattress to raise her up. Lying flat makes the cough much worse. Coughs are also often exacerbated by dry air. At night, put a bowl of boiling water (out of reach) containing a few drops of lavender and eucalyptus essential oils in your child's room. This will help to ease

the breathing, especially if the nose and chest are congested with mucus. For croup and recurrent chest infections, an electric humidifier will also help to provide relief from the symptoms.

Medicinal foods for coughs

If the cough accompanies a cold, there are dietary strategies that you can follow to help your child combat the viral infection and ease the symptoms. Cold viruses often stimulate an over-production of mucus that leaves your child feeling "blocked up" and uncomfortable. To avoid making this worse, eliminate mucus-forming foods, especially dairy products, from their diet. This includes milk, cream, yoghurt, ice cream and cheese. Other foods that tend to increase mucus production and are therefore best avoided include egg, fried foods, red meat and foods containing sugar or excessive salt.

Foods that help to break down mucus are citrus fruits, garlic and onion, celery, parsley, chicken broth, chilli peppers, watercress, horseradish and green tea. Offer your child a hot toddy of lemon and honey and prepare an immune-boosting chicken broth (see page 126) to aid the healing process. Encourage her to drink plenty of fluids as this helps to thin the mucus, which in turn makes it easier to cough up. Make fresh juices from fruits and vegetables that are full of antioxidants, which will help your child to fight the infection. If your child's throat is very sore offer antioxidant-rich ice pops, which will help to soothe and anaesthetize the throat. Blackcurrants and strawberries are especially rich in antioxidant vitamins and phytonutrients and make absolutely delicious ice pops (see page 125).

Include plenty of vitamin C and beta-carotene in your child's diet if she is suffering from a cough, as these are key antioxidants and will help her immune cells to fight the infection. Foods that are particularly good sources of vitamin C include citrus fruits, peppers and kiwi fruit. As well as having antioxidant properties, vitamin C is anti-inflammatory and therefore very useful when treating an inflamed and sore upper respiratory tract. It can also boost the production of interferon, an antiviral agent that enhances the ability of the respiratory tract to ward off viruses. Beta-carotene is the plant-based form of vitamin A and is needed to protect the mucous membranes. Vitamin A is also found in animal-based foods, such as eggs and liver, but as these tend to be mucus forming, it is far better to prepare your child dishes that include good sources of beta-carotene. Fruits and vegetables rich in

beta-carotene are brightly coloured and include carrots, sweet potatoes and green leafy vegetables.

Foods rich in zinc are also important in the fight against respiratory infection. Research has shown that zinc can cut the occurrence of acute respiratory infections by almost half. Good sources are poultry, game, seeds, nuts, seafood and wholegrains.

Avoid sugary foods, which are immune-suppressive, and refined foods such as white flour and white rice. These foods have had important nutrients stripped out of them during the refining process and may simply serve to fill up your child without supplying her with any of the nutrients that can help to aid her recovery.

Warming herbs and spices can be soothing and effective for coughs. Garlic and thyme have excellent antiviral and antibacterial properties. Ginger, cloves and cinnamon all have expectorant qualities that help to expel the mucus. Thyme and honey tea can be comforting and calming to a tickly cough (see below). Manuka (tea tree) honey is a particularly good addition as it contains natural antibiotic properties.

SUGGESTED RECIPES FOR COUGHS

clove tea
🔲🔲🔲🔲 🔲1⁺2⁺5⁺

1 cup (225 ml/8 fl oz) boiling water
2–3 cloves
1 tsp Manuka honey

Pour the water over the cloves and leave to steep for 10 minutes. Remove the cloves, add the honey and tell your child to sip slowly for a comforting winter-warming tonic for the chest.

thyme and honey tea
🔲🔲🔲🔲 🔲1⁺2⁺5⁺

1 tsp fresh thyme leaves
1 cup (225 ml/8 fl oz) boiling water
Juice of 1 lemon
1–2 tsp Manuka honey

Place the thyme in a teapot and cover with the boiling water. Add the lemon juice and honey and stir well. Allow to sit for 3–4 minutes. Strain the tea into a cup and tell your child to drink slowly.

thyme and chicken casserole
🔲🔲🔲🔲 🔲1⁺2⁺5⁺

1 chicken
2 garlic cloves, peeled
3–4 sprigs of thyme
1 carrot, peeled and chopped
1 sweet potato, peeled and chopped
10 shallots, peeled
1 litre (1¾ pints) apple juice

Preheat the oven to 190°C/350°F/Gas Mark 4. Place the chicken in a casserole dish and surround it with the garlic, thyme and all of the vegetables. Pour over the apple juice so that it comes half way up the chicken. Bake in the oven for 1½ hours until the chicken is cooked through. Transfer the chicken to a serving plate. Remove the thyme and any excess fat from the casserole. With a slotted spoon, scoop out the vegetables and shallots and lay them around the bottom of the chicken. Bring the remaining liquid to the boil, and continue boiling for a few minutes to reduce it to a gravy. Pour the gravy over the chicken and serve with a green vegetable such as broccoli or kale.

chicken pox

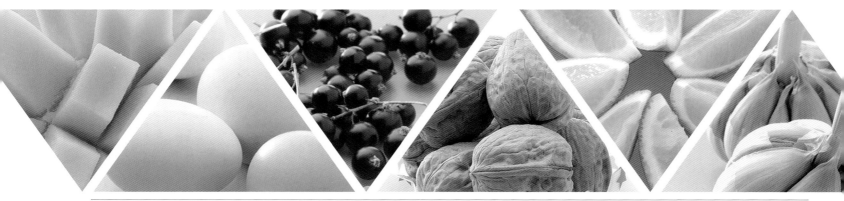

STAR FOODS FOR CHICKEN POX: ALMOND, APRICOT, BEETROOT, BLACKCURRANT, BLUEBERRY, BUTTERNUT SQUASH, CANTALOUPE MELON, CARROT, CASHEW NUT, CINNAMON, CITRUS FRUITS, EGG, GARLIC, GINGER, GUAVA, KIWI FRUIT, MANGO, OATS, ONION, PAPAYA, PARSLEY, PUMPKIN SEED, RASPBERRY, STRAWBERRY, SUNFLOWER SEED, SWEET POTATO, TOFU, WALNUT

Chicken pox is a highly infectious childhood disease caused by the varicella-zoster virus from the herpes family. Most children will contract chicken pox at some time during their childhood as it is spread very easily through coughing, sneezing and even talking. The incubation period for the disease is two weeks and a child with chicken pox is contagious for one to two days before any of the symptoms appear until all the spots have scabbed over. This usually takes between nine and 12 days.

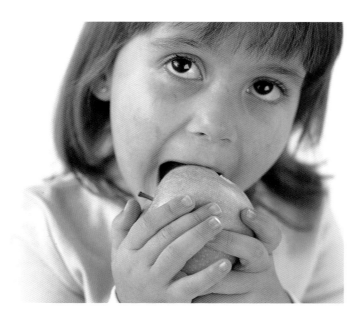

The first symptom of chicken pox is usually a fever, sometimes accompanied by a headache. Your child will not feel well, as with any virus. After a day or two, little blisters begin to appear, starting on the chest and back and then spreading to the rest of the body. A child or baby with very mild chicken pox may get only a few of them. Equally, a particularly aggressive strain can cause hundreds of spots all over the body as well as in the mouth, ears, eyes and bottom. In families where there are several siblings, the child who contracts chicken pox first is likely to get the mildest dose. As it is passed on to another child, the symptoms become more aggressive. During the eruptive phase of chicken pox, each and every individual spot can be extremely itchy.

Medicinal foods for chicken pox

Certain foods can be highly beneficial for children suffering from chicken pox, especially during the healing process. A child who has contracted the virus needs to have their immune system replenished and bolstered and you need to pay special attention to foods containing nutrients that help repair damaged skin. While your child is in the middle of the illness and has itchy spots, baths with ½ cup of bicarbonate of soda added help to relieve the itching and can be taken several times a day. Chicken pox can leave scars, especially if your child scratches the spots a great deal. Supplying your child with foods rich in beta-carotene, vitamin C and flavonoids will help in the healing of skin tissue and the mucous membranes often damaged by the virus. A recent study showed that chicken pox can deplete a child's vitamin A levels for several months. Including plenty of orange, red, and dark green vegetables and fruit in your child's diet will ensure that she is receiving plenty of beta-carotene, the plant form of vitamin A, which her body can then convert into the crucial vitamin at her own requirement level. Retinol, which is the active form of vitamin A found in animal-based foods such as egg, liver and dairy products, can be toxic in excess. Therefore, boosting beta-carotene levels in very young children is always the safest option when trying to increase their levels of vitamin A.

A child with chicken pox will not often feel like eating much, so preparing fresh juices and smoothies made from some of the fruits and vegetables listed under the star foods for chicken pox (left) will supply plenty of antioxidants to help in the healing process.

Some children get chicken pox in their throats. If this is the case with your child, try giving her fresh fruit juice ice pops, which can be very comforting. You can use any fruits or fruit juices for this but blackcurrants are particularly good as they are full of both vitamin C, which helps to fight the infection and repair the skin, and anthocyanins, phytonutrients that multiply vitamin C's antioxidant power as well as having anti-inflammatory properties. Try the recipe for blackcurrant and strawberry ice pops on page 125.

Making sure that your child drinks plenty of fluids is vital, as this will prevent dehydration, especially if a fever is present. Offering water bottles and juices through straws or from a teaspoon may help to encourage your young child or baby to take in fluid. For babies over the age of six months who are no longer being breastfed, avoid dairy formulas if a fever is present and offer almond or rice milks during the acute phase of the illness instead. Infants who are still being breastfed will receive plenty of immune-boosting substances through the breast milk.

During the illness prepare meals that are rich in nutrients and low in sugar, saturated fat and salt. Do not be tempted to give your child sweets, chocolate or sugar-laden yoghurts in an attempt to get them to eat something. Sick children rarely want to eat and enticing them to eat such foods will only further suppress their immune systems. Once your child starts to feel better, complement

the drinks by offering comforting soups and broths. Include plenty of garlic, which contains antiviral substances. Nuts and seeds offered as snacks or as part of a meal are a good source of energy and are rich in essential fatty acids, zinc and B-vitamins, all of which aid the healing process.

Echinacea and golden seal are two herbs that can help fight the infection and strengthen your child's immune defences. Golden seal is also antipyretic (fever reducing) so is additionally beneficial. These two herbs can be found in health food shops and are easily added to drinks in tincture form at an appropriate dosage for age.

SUGGESTED RECIPES FOR CHICKEN POX

blueberry smoothie
serves one

1 cup (225 ml/8 fl oz) apple juice
2 ripe bananas
1 cup (115 g/4 oz) blueberries
1 tbsp linseed oil
1 cup (115 g/4 oz) raspberries

Liquidize all the ingredients together in a blender. Serve immediately with a straw.

chicken noodle soup
serves two

1 garlic clove, crushed
1 onion, chopped
1 tbsp extra virgin olive oil
1 skinless and boneless chicken breast, cubed
3 carrots, diced
600 ml (1 pint) vegetable stock
1 handful of rice noodles
1 tbsp chopped parsley

Gently sauté the garlic and onion in the olive oil until transparent. Add the chicken breast and cook for 3–4 minutes. Add the carrots and stock. Cover and gently simmer for 15 minutes. Meanwhile, soak the rice noodles in some boiling water for 5 minutes. Once the chicken is cooked through, drain the noodles and add them to the soup along with the chopped parsley. Cover and leave to cool slightly for 5–10 minutes. The noodles will swell up to create a thick soup that children will enjoy and find easy to eat.

chronic fatigue syndrome

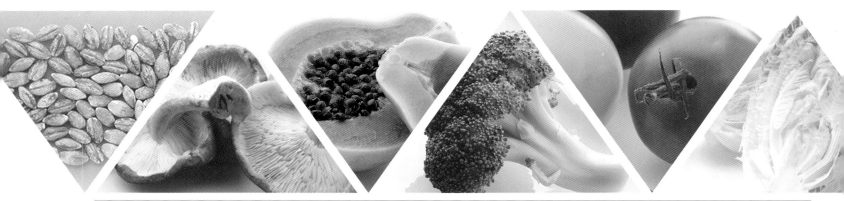

STAR FOODS FOR CHRONIC FATIGUE SYNDROME: APRICOT, AVOCADO, BANANA, BARLEY, BEANSPROUT, BEETROOT, BLACKCURRANT, BLUEBERRY, BROCCOLI, BROWN RICE, BUTTERNUT SQUASH, CARROT, DUCK, EGG, FRESH TUNA, GARLIC, KALE, KIWI FRUIT, LETTUCE, MANGO, ORANGE, PAPAYA, PARSLEY, SALMON, SHIITAKE MUSHROOM, SWEET POTATO, TOMATO, VENISON

Exactly how chronic fatigue syndrome (also known as myalgic encephalomyelitis, or ME) develops is not known, nor is there any cure for the condition at present. However, most sufferers do recover over time. There has been great controversy over CFS in the medical profession, and it was not until the mid-1990s that doctors agreed to make the diagnosis if there were a number of specific symptoms present.

Chronic fatigue syndrome rarely affects children before their teens. It is more common in females than males and appears to be more likely to occur where there is a family history of allergies. CFS can often be traced back to a viral infection from which the sufferer never properly recovered. This could simply be the flu or, more commonly, another virus such as Epstein-Barr, a member of the herpes group of viruses, which is responsible for glandular fever. It has been found that 40 per cent of CFS sufferers are infected with the Epstein-Barr virus. One characteristic common to the herpes group of viruses is their ability to lay dormant after the initial infection. A healthy immune system will keep this dormant virus in check but, if the immune system is compromised, the virus can be reactivated.

In an attempt to define the disease, researchers in Australia proposed a table of symptoms that is now widely recognized to help in the diagnosis. The three major signs of CFS are:
- Fatigue – either intermittent or persistent, which has lasted for longer than six months and is made worse through exercise
- Mental impairment, such as poor concentration and short-term memory loss
- Decreased immune function with a reduction of the body's white blood cell count

Other supporting symptoms might include muscle and joint pain with swelling and tenderness, headaches, sore throat, tinnitus, enlarged glands, insomnia and irritable bowel syndrome.

Medicinal foods for chronic fatigue syndrome

If your child does contract chronic fatigue syndrome, the focus must be on building up the strength of her immune system. Start by eliminating any foods that are likely to put an additional burden on the body. Processed children's meals and snacks, laden with chemical additives, will only further tax an already depleted immune system. Foods high in sugar, colours and artificial sweeteners, such as fizzy drinks, jellies and sweets, are another source of strain. A good diet for chronic fatigue syndrome consists of fruits, vegetables, grains, lean meat and fish. Rather than large, heavy meals, try making soups, smoothies, juices and broths that are easy to eat and supply all of the nutrients required to assist recovery.

Focus on foods that will help to fight the virus. Garlic has strong antiviral properties and can be a useful addition to your child's diet. Foods full of vitamin C also display antiviral properties by enhancing white blood cell activity. White blood cells are the key fighters in the immune army and work to engulf and destroy viruses. Vitamin C-rich foods include citrus fruits, kiwi fruit, guava, peppers and blackcurrants. Beta-carotene is another nutrient that demonstrates antiviral properties. It can stimulate white blood cell production and enhances the activity of interferon, an antiviral protein created by the body to help contain the spread of disease. Foods rich in beta-carotene are brightly coloured, especially red and orange fruits and vegetables such as carrots, apricots, mango, papaya, tomatoes, peppers, sweet potatoes and squash. In addition, vitamin C and beta-carotene are powerful antioxidants, which means that they give a general boost to the immune system by mopping up harmful free radicals.

The shiitake mushroom has long been used in traditional Chinese medicine to enhance resistance to disease and to fight viruses. It contains the immune-boosting phytonutrient lentinan, which appears to be able to prevent virus replication as well as induce interferon production.

If your child is diagnosed as being infected by the Epstein-Barr virus, there are specific additional dietary measures you can take to help. The Epstein-Barr virus is nourished by an amino acid called arginine, which is found in large concentrations in beans and nuts. However, arginine has a natural antidote in the form of another amino acid, lysine, which prevents arginine's viral-nourishing effects. A diet high in lysine and low in arginine has been shown to help prevent recurrent infections caused by the herpes family of viruses. Foods high in lysine are eggs, cheese, fish and poultry. Arginine-rich foods are chocolate, beans, nuts and tofu, and are best avoided.

Chronic fatigue sufferers have been shown to have low supplies of magnesium in their bodies. Magnesium is required for energy production as well as muscle function and low levels can cause general as well as muscle fatigue. Offer broths, stews and stir-fries containing plenty of magnesium-rich foods, such as green leafy vegetables and wholegrains, to help redress this imbalance.

SUGGESTED RECIPES FOR CFS

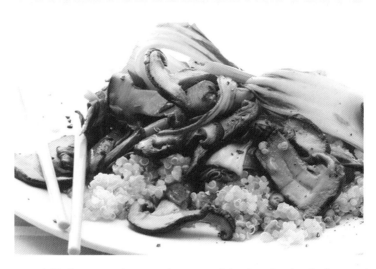

shiitake, spring onion and bok choi stir-fry with quinoa

🗷🗷🗷🖊 🖊1⁺2⁺5⁺ serves one

¼ cup (60 g/2 oz) quinoa, washed
A handful of spring onions, washed and sliced
1 tbsp extra virgin olive oil
10 shiitake mushrooms, washed and sliced
2 stalks bok choi, washed and sliced
1 garlic clove, chopped
1 tbsp tamari (wheat-free) soy sauce

Bring a saucepan of water to the boil, add the quinoa and gently simmer for 15–20 minutes until cooked. Meanwhile, in a wok, cook the spring onions in the olive oil for a couple of minutes. Add the shiitake mushrooms, bok choi and garlic and continue to stir-fry for 1 minute. Toss in the tamari and stir-fry for a further couple of minutes. Drain the cooked quinoa and serve with the stir-fry on top.

carrot and onion soup

🗷🗷🗷🖊 🖊1⁺2⁺5⁺

1 tbsp extra virgin olive oil
1 garlic clove, crushed
1 onion, finely chopped
1 bag of carrots, chopped
600 ml (1 pint) vegetable stock
A few sprigs of parsley
Live natural yoghurt to serve (optional)

In a saucepan, heat the oil and cook the garlic and onion until translucent. Add the carrots and the stock and simmer gently for 25 minutes until the carrots are soft. Liquidize the soup with the parsley until smooth. Serve plain or dressed with a dollop of live natural yoghurt.

eczema

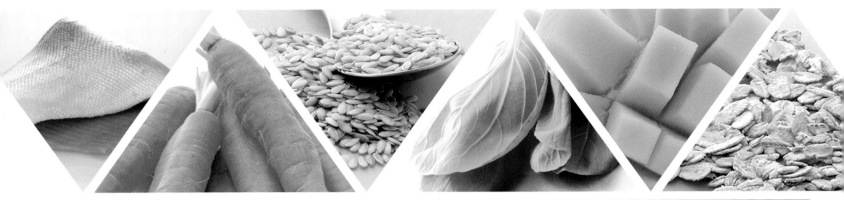

STAR FOODS FOR ECZEMA: ALMOND, APPLE CIDER VINEGAR, APRICOT, AVOCADO, BREAST MILK, BUTTERNUT SQUASH, CANTALOUPE MELON, CARROT, EVENING PRIMROSE OIL, FRESH TUNA, GAME, GREEN LEAFY VEGETABLES, HERRING, LINSEED (FLAXSEED) OIL, MACKEREL, MANGO, NUTS, OATS, PUMPKIN AND PUMPKIN SEED, SALMON, SEEDS AND THEIR OILS, SUNFLOWER SEED, SWEET POTATO

Eczema is an inflammatory skin condition characterized by areas of dry, flaky, red and itchy patches of skin. It is extremely common in young children, with as many as one in four of those under eight years old suffering. It is also called dermatitis and comes in several varieties. The most common form is atopic eczema, which is more often found in families with a history of allergic conditions such as asthma, hay fever, migraine or eczema itself. This type of eczema often starts in the transition from breast to bottle or when solids are first introduced. Children with atopic eczema usually grow out of the condition by the age of 15. Other types of eczema include nummular dermatitis, often triggered by a nickel allergy, causing circular, scaly lesions on the limbs. Dermatitis herpetiformis is a very itchy form of eczema and often accompanies bowel disorders. It is thought to be triggered by consumption of gluten and/or dairy products. Seborrhoeic eczema commonly affects the scalp and face.

Eczema can be triggered by a wide range of potential irritants, such as house dust mites, pets, soaps and detergents, bubble baths, shampoos, chlorine, food allergies, wool and synthetic fibres. Stress and viral infections can exacerbate symptoms. If you suspect that your child has eczema as a result of a food allergy, try undertaking an exclusion diet, with the assistance of a qualified nutritionist, in order to identify, and then avoid, the culprits.

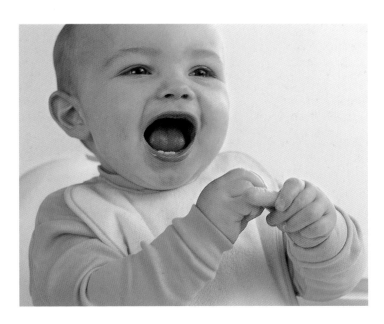

Medicinal foods for eczema

Eczema often appears in the transitional period of weaning. If your family has a history of allergies, or your baby shows signs of eczema, delay introducing solids until six months of age. Breastfeeding provides protection against allergies owing to the unique nutritional profile of the breast milk. Early exposure to foods increases the likelihood of allergic reactions owing to the baby's undeveloped digestive system. When you do start weaning, begin with fresh fruit and vegetable purées, progressing to rice, millet and other grains, beans and pulses, seeds, fish and poultry. Avoid cow's milk, egg, wheat, tomato and citrus fruits until after the age of one.

Essential fatty acids (EFAs) are vital components of your child's diet, as every cell in their body requires them. They are also anti-inflammatory so can be used in treating eczema. Breast milk is a rich source of EFAs, whereas an infant diet of dairy and commercial baby foods contains very little. To incorporate EFAs into your child's diet, you can add a teaspoon of linseed (flaxseed) oil to your baby's food once a day from the age of six months. Other good EFA food sources are safflower oil, sunflower seeds and their oils, pumpkin seeds, evening primrose oil, walnuts and oily fish. Some EFA sources can also be administered externally. If your child has eczema, rub the contents of a 500 mg capsule of evening primrose oil into her tummy or inner thighs (wherever there is no eczema) up to six times a day.

Eczema sufferers tend to have low levels of certain nutrients including zinc, magnesium, B-vitamins and vitamin C. If your child develops eczema, it may be worthwhile to ask a nutritional therapist or doctor who practises complementary medicine to carry out a sweat test or hair-mineral analysis test (both non-invasive) to establish mineral levels. You can then incorporate foods rich in any of the minerals your child is lacking into her diet.

Foods rich in the antioxidants beta-carotene, vitamin E and selenium are all important for skin healing. Include lots of red and orange fruits and vegetables, as well as nuts and seeds and their oils, in the diet to provide plenty of these nutrients.

A great remedy for itchy skin is to add ½ cup of apple cider vinegar and ⅓ cup of cold-pressed oil (try sunflower) to your child's bath. Pat your child dry to retain some of the oil on her skin.

SUGGESTED RECIPES FOR ECZEMA

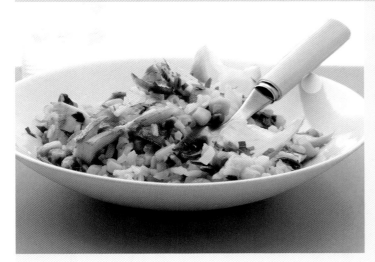

almond milk

🗙🗙🗙✎   ✐1⁺2⁺5⁺   makes one glass or beaker

Almond milk is a dairy-free source of protein, calcium and magnesium.

½ cup (75 g/2¾ oz) blanched almonds
½ cup (115 ml/4 fl oz) filtered water
1 tsp Manuka honey
1 tbsp essential balance oil (an EFA blend available in health food shops)

To blanch the almonds, place them in a sieve and dip them in boiling water for about half a minute. The skins will then pop off easily. Put the almonds and the water in a liquidizer and blend until smooth. Add the honey and essential balance oil and blend again. Sieve the mixture to remove any lumps and serve immediately. Add a chopped, frozen banana to make a more creamy shake.

salmon kedgeree

🗙🗙🗙✎   ✐1⁺2⁺5⁺

1 skinless and boneless salmon fillet
1 onion, chopped
1 tbsp extra virgin olive oil
1 cup (200 g/7 oz) brown rice
A handful of frozen peas
1 tin of sweetcorn (no-sugar, no-salt variety)
A little unhydrogenated vegetable margarine (or butter if dairy-tolerant)
A small handful of finely chopped parsley

Preheat the oven to 190°C/375°F/Gas Mark 5. Bake the salmon fillet in the oven for 20 minutes until cooked through. Flake the fish and place in a serving dish. Gently cook the onion in the olive oil until soft. Add this to the serving dish. Meanwhile, cook the rice in a pan of boiling water for 35–40 minutes until soft. Drain well and add to the fish mixture. Lightly steam the peas for 5 minutes, adding the corn at the last minute to heat through. Add this to the fish and rice. Mix everything together well and dot the top of the dish with butter or unhydrogenated margarine. Bake in the oven for 20 minutes and sprinkle with the parsley before serving.

food allergies

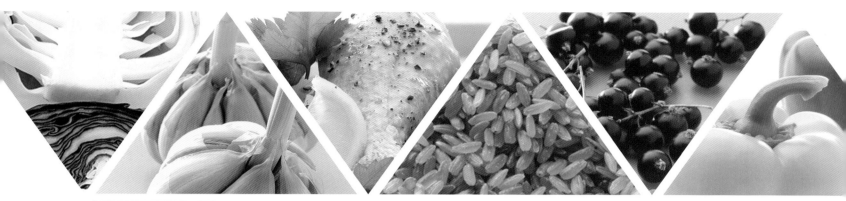

STAR FOODS FOR ALLERGIES: ALMOND, APPLE, APRICOT, BLACKCURRANT, BLUEBERRY, BOK CHOI, BROCCOLI, BROWN RICE, BUCKWHEAT, BUTTERNUT SQUASH, CABBAGE, CANTALOUPE MELON, CARROT, GAME, GARLIC, KALE, MILLET, ONION, PEAR, PEPPERS, PUMPKIN AND PUMPKIN SEED, QUINOA, SALMON, SUNFLOWER SEED, SWEET POTATO

Allergies are becoming increasingly common in the Western world. Symptoms range from a constant runny nose to full-blown anaphylactic shock, which can cause death. Allergens, the substances that cause allergies, can come from the environment, such as pollen, dust and mould, or from foods, such as nuts. The same symptoms can be caused by different allergens. Similarly, individuals can react in different ways to the same allergens.

It is now estimated that as many as one in five children in the UK suffers from the allergic illnesses eczema and asthma. The countries with the highest rates of asthma in the world are the UK, Australia, New Zealand and the US. The places with the lowest asthma rates are the Mediterranean countries, Eastern Europe and India. The question of why there has been such a rapid escalation of the problem in some countries in recent years is still subject to speculative debate. Some blame poor diet and environmental pollution. There is certainly no doubt that environmental pollution plays a part and that a diet low in antioxidants and vitamins will make a child more susceptible to allergies. However, introducing solid food to a baby too early can also increase the risk of allergies.

Another suggested explanation for the general increase in children suffering from allergies is the hygiene hypothesis. This states that our children's immune systems are not being primed as they used to be while very young because of our obsession with cleanliness and germ avoidance in the developed world. Whatever the reasons, allergy prevention has to be the focus for the parents of the future. Genetic inheritance does play a crucial role but there are ways, through diet, in which parents can delay and reduce the symptoms of allergies and intolerances should their children be susceptible to them.

Food allergy or intolerance?

The issue of whether your child is suffering from a food allergy or a food intolerance adds controversy and confusion to the allergy debate. A food allergy is defined by an immediate immune response. When food allergens enter your child's body, her immune system reacts by producing large amounts of the chemical histamine. It is the release of histamine that results in the allergic reaction with its recognizable symptoms. These are usually first noted in the facial area, with an itchiness around the mouth or swelling in the lips. This can be accompanied by a severe stomach ache, nausea, diarrhoea and/or rashes. Occasionally it can result in difficulty breathing, in which case urgent medical attention is required. The same common foods cause most of these allergic reactions: milk, wheat, eggs, soya products, fish, shellfish, nuts and sesame seeds.

A food intolerance manifests itself in a different way. Although there may be an immune response, this is not always the case. More often an intolerance appears as a delayed response to foods frequently eaten and is, therefore, far more difficult to detect or isolate. Symptoms of food intolerance include asthma, eczema, hyperactivity, migraine, skin rashes, glue ear, persistent runny nose, stomach aches, vomiting and diarrhoea, insomnia, bed wetting, fatigue, and aching muscles and joints. Food intolerances often occur in reaction to the foods most frequently eaten. Common offenders in this category are milk and wheat. Offering your baby or child a varied diet rather than relying too heavily on one or two basic foods is the best protection you can provide against intolerances.

Preventing allergies and intolerances in older children

After the age of one, your baby should be eating the same meals as the rest of the family. The golden rule for protecting children of all ages against allergies and intolerances is to provide plenty of variety in their diet. Intolerances are most likely to occur when foods are served up repetitively in different guises. For example, if a child is eating cereal with milk and toast for breakfast, followed by a pasta dish for lunch and sandwiches and yoghurts for tea, their diet consists predominantly of wheat and dairy – two of the most common triggers for allergies and intolerances. Experimenting with a variety of grains and dairy alternatives will prevent this from occurring. If you were to offer porridge for breakfast or a boiled egg with rye toast soldiers, followed by a rice dish at lunch and sandwiches for tea, you would only have used wheat once in the day and provided a much greater variety of nutrients.

If, however, your child is already showing symptoms of intolerance or allergy, remove the suspect food or food group for a month and see if the symptoms improve. If they do, the food can sometimes be gradually reintroduced to the diet in small amounts and your child may develop a level of tolerance for it. Strict food elimination diets involving more than one food or a food group should be carried out only under the guidance of a healthcare professional. This ensures that you are using suitable alternatives to these foods and food groups which will supply your child with all the nutrients that she requires.

For an allergic child, prepare foods rich in the anti-allergenic nutrients and antioxidants that support the immune system

generally. The essential fatty acids found in evening primrose oil, linseed (flaxseed) oil and fish oils can be beneficial (as long as the allergy is not to fish) as these help to regulate and control the inflammatory response. Foods rich in vitamin C, beta-carotene, flavonoids (especially quercetin), zinc, magnesium and calcium all help to protect your child against allergies because they contain a combination of antioxidant, anti-inflammatory and antihistamine properties. See the list of star foods for allergies (left) for foods to include in your child's diet.

PROTECTING BABIES AGAINST ALLERGIES

Until your baby reaches the age of six months, the best protection you can give her against developing allergies of any kind is to feed her a diet of breast milk only. Once she is six months old, start the weaning process (see page 68) but use this chart to see which foods are best avoided until a later stage so that they don't overburden an immature digestive system and trigger an allergy or intolerance. The foods marked with an asterix are those that can cause allergic type reactions.

6 months
At this age your baby can eat:
- All vegetables except those listed under 9 months
- All fruits except those listed under 9 and 12 months
- Dried fruits (unsulphured)
- Non-gluten grains: rice, millet, buckwheat, quinoa
- Beans and pulses (except soya beans)
- Organic poultry, game and meat
- Fish* (except shellfish)

9 months
At this age your baby can eat:
- Potatoes, tomatoes, aubergines, peppers
- Gluten grains: oats, barley, rye, semolina (occasionally), corn
- Soya products*
- Ground nuts* and seeds*
- Egg yolks

12 months
At this age your baby can eat:
- Citrus fruit
- Dairy products: milk*, yoghurt, cheese
- Wheat: bread, pasta, flour
- Whole eggs*

2 years
At this age your child can eat:
- Strawberries
- Shellfish*

5 years
At this age your child can eat:
- Whole nuts*

In addition you should avoid feeding your baby the following foods altogether, and keep them to an absolute minimum as your child grows up:
- Salt
- Additives found in processed foods and drinks
- Hydrogenated fat
- Stimulants, such as caffeine

glandular fever

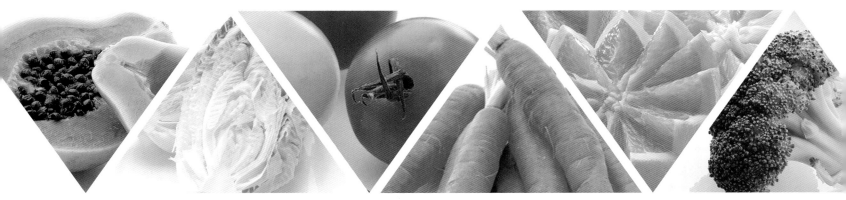

STAR FOODS FOR GLANDULAR FEVER: APRICOT, AVOCADO, BANANA, BARLEY, BEANSPROUT, BEETROOT, BLACKCURRANT, BLUEBERRY, BROCCOLI, BROWN RICE, BUTTERNUT SQUASH, CARROT, DUCK, FRESH TUNA, GARLIC, KALE, KIWI FRUIT, LETTUCE, MANGO, ORANGE, PAPAYA, PARSLEY, PUMPKIN SEED, SALMON, SHIITAKE MUSHROOM, SUNFLOWER SEED, SWEET POTATO, TOMATO, VENISON

Glandular fever (also called mononucleosis) is a viral infection caused in the majority of cases by the Epstein-Barr virus, a member of the herpes family. Although it can occur in very young children, it is most common during the teenage years. The virus is transmitted through saliva and has earned the nickname of the "kissing disease". Diagnosis of this viral infection is confirmed by a blood test, followed by liver function tests if necessary.

Symptoms include a fever, swollen glands, sore throat, aching muscles, overwhelming fatigue, an enlarged spleen and abnormal liver function. A child with glandular fever is likely to be very weak and tired. In young children, the virus usually lasts from two to four weeks. In older children, however, it can last up to several months. To prevent any damage to the liver and spleen, bed-rest is essential during the initial stages of the illness.

Medicinal foods for glandular fever

To aid recovery from glandular fever, particular attention to diet is essential. Give your child plenty of water and diluted fruit juices to help flush out toxins from the body. Water supports the lymphatic system (see page 11), a critical part of your child's immune system, by stopping it from becoming sluggish. If a fever is present, frequent fluids are important to stop your child from becoming dehydrated. If your child's throat is particularly sore, small, frequent sips are often the least painful way for her to drink liquids. Fresh

fruit juice ice pops can also be useful in helping to ease the discomfort and supplying fluid at the same time.

A child with glandular fever should follow a diet consisting of fruits, vegetables, grains, lean meat and fish. While the appetite is suppressed as a result of the illness, offer lighter meals of soups, smoothies, juices and broths that will be easy to eat and will provide a good supply of the nutrients needed to assist recovery. As the liver may be compromised by the virus, it is wise to avoid

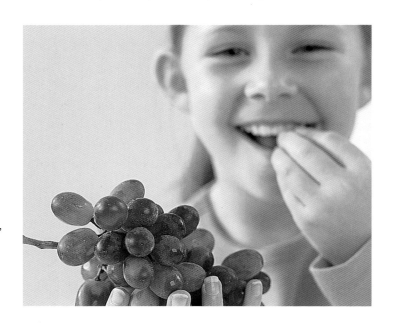

unnecessary fat in the diet because one of the functions of the liver is to secrete bile in order to break down food fats. A weakened liver needs all the help it can get, and cutting down on fats will avoid over-taxing it. Foods containing sugar and refined flour should also be kept to a minimum as they are immune-suppressive. Cut out soft drinks, processed and fried foods, all of which depress immunity.

During the recovery period you should prepare foods for your child that are rich in the antioxidant vitamins A, C and E. This will help boost her immune system to fight the infection. Vitamin C is also essential for the production of antibodies and interferon, both of which play key roles in combating and destroying the cells of a viral infection. Vitamin C is a water-soluble vitamin and cannot be stored by the body. It therefore needs to be acquired through diet on a daily basis. Foods particularly rich in vitamin C are citrus fruits, peppers, kiwi fruit, blackcurrants and guava.

The best way to incorporate vitamin A into your child's diet is to offer foods containing beta-carotene. This is an antioxidant carotenoid and is the plant-based form of vitamin A which can be converted into the vitamin by your child's body as and when needed. In addition, beta-carotene has antiviral properties, helping to stimulate the production and activity of white blood cells. Foods rich in beta-carotene include apricot, mango, cantaloupe melon, tomato, carrot, butternut squash, other squashes and sweet potato.

Vitamin E, a fat-soluble vitamin that the body can store, is required for the health and maintenance of all cells and body tissue as well as for its antioxidant qualities. As such, it helps to repair cells damaged by the virus and boosts the immune system to fight free radicals, which also cause cell damage. It can be found in such foods as avocado, butternut squash, seeds and seed oils.

Studies have shown that the Epstein-Barr virus that causes glandular fever is strengthened by the amino acid arginine. This is found in chocolate, nuts and seeds, beans and tofu, so these foods should be avoided. However, another amino acid, lysine, has been found to be able to operate as an antibody to arginine. Thus, a diet high in lysine and low in arginine has been shown to help prevent recurrent infections caused by the herpes family of viruses. Foods rich in lysine include eggs, cheese, fish and poultry.

Two particular star foods to include in the diet of a child with glandular fever are shiitake mushrooms and garlic. The shiitake mushroom has been used in traditional Chinese medicine for many centuries in the battle against disease and to fight viruses. Its magical property is lentinan, an immune-boosting phytonutrient that appears to be able to prevent virus replication. Lentinan also induces interferon production, which further helps the body to fight off infection. Make sure to use plenty of garlic in your child's diet – it is a potent antiviral and can be easily added to many meals.

SUGGESTED RECIPES FOR GLANDULAR FEVER

guava smoothie

serves one

1 banana, peeled
½ cup (115 ml/4 fl oz) fresh apple juice
1 guava, peeled
½ cup (150 ml/5 fl oz) natural yoghurt (optional)

Liquidize the ingredients together in a blender and serve.

energy salad with garlic and honey dressing

serves one

A few assorted leafy green salad leaves
1 small carrot, peeled and grated
A small handful of raisins
A small handful of bean sprouts
A few slices of cucumber
A handful of sunflower seeds, toasted
A couple of cherry tomatoes, halved

Arrange the above decoratively in a bowl and pour over the dressing.

GARLIC AND HONEY DRESSING
1 garlic clove, crushed
1 tsp runny honey
1 tsp Dijon mustard
1 tbsp apple cider vinegar
2 tbsp linseed oil or extra virgin olive oil

Mix together the garlic, honey and mustard and then add the apple cider vinegar and the oil and mix well.

hay fever

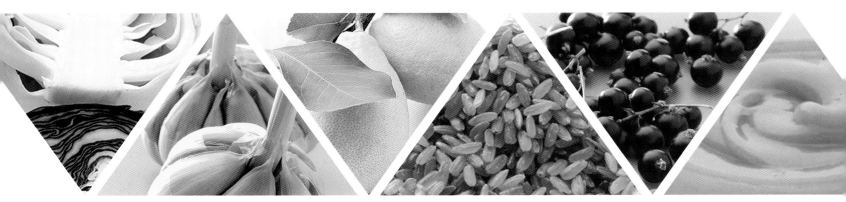

STAR FOODS FOR HAY FEVER: ALMOND, BARLEY, BLACKBERRY, BLACKCURRANT, BLUEBERRY, BROCCOLI, BROWN RICE, BUCKWHEAT, CABBAGE, FIG, GARLIC, GINGER, GRAPEFRUIT, HONEY, HORSERADISH, KALE, LEMON, LIME, MACKEREL, ONION, ORANGE, ROCKET, ROSEMARY, SALMON, SARDINE, THYME, TURMERIC, TURNIP, WATERCRESS

Hay fever (or allergic rhinitis, also known as seasonal rhinitis) is a seasonal allergy. It is caused by pollens produced by trees and grasses in spring and summer. Hay fever often runs in families, especially where there is a history of other allergic diseases such as eczema and asthma. In a child, hay fever is most likely to manifest itself after the age of six years and, today, as many as one in ten adults suffer from the disease in one form or another.

Hay fever symptoms are caused by an immune response to pollen that causes the mucous membranes in the nasal cavity to become inflamed. When pollen comes into contact with the membranes, the immune system goes on the assault and creates antibodies to it. If children are not allergic to pollen, this response is a normal, low-key one and goes unnoticed. If, however, your child has a pollen allergy, an extreme response is triggered, resulting in a mass production of histamine and other inflammatory chemicals that, in turn, cause the symptoms of hay fever. These include sneezing, itchy and watering eyes, runny nose, itchy and sore throat, swollen eyes and itchy and irritated skin. Sufferers are also likely to feel tired, irritable and have difficulty concentrating.

Medicinal foods for hay fever

If your child does suffer from hay fever it is advisable to remove dairy products from her diet during the hay fever season. This includes milk, cream, cheese, yoghurt and ice cream. Dairy products increase mucus production and are a common allergen during childhood. Replace them with other sources of calcium and protein, such as nuts and seeds, beans, fortified soya products, fortified rice drinks, green leafy vegetables and molasses.

Another food that may exacerbate hay fever is wheat. This is originally a grass product and, although no formal studies have yet been carried out, it is suggested that some hay fever sufferers become hypersensitive to the proteins that are common in wheat and other grasses. Another consideration is that intensive farming practices mean that today's wheat is much higher in gluten, a common gut irritant which stimulates mucus production. A simple month's exclusion will help to identify if wheat is indeed worsening your child's hay fever. Alternatives to common wheat products include rye breads and crackers, oats and oat cakes, gluten-free flours, brown rice, millet, quinoa and buckwheat.

Give your child foods rich in beta-carotene to help reduce allergic reactions and soothe mucous membranes. Beta-carotene can be found in all yellow, orange and red fruits, and in vegetables such as carrot, peppers, pumpkin, squash and sweet potato.

Phytonutrients from the flavonoid group, especially quercetin, are known for their antihistamine qualities. Quercetin is found in the peel of citrus fruits as well as in buckwheat, coloured onions, apple, tomato, potato, grapes and broad beans. It also enhances the body's absorption of vitamin C, another antihistamine. These two substances are often found together in foods, a common example being citrus fruits. Other vitamin C-rich foods include blackcurrants, kiwi fruit, guava and peppers.

Garlic can also provide relief for hay fever sufferers as it helps to reduce sinus inflammation. Include plenty in stir-fries, soups and salad dressings. Other herbs and spices that can help relieve the symptoms of hay fever are horseradish, chilli, ginger, cinnamon and turmeric, all of which have decongestant and expectorant qualities.

Calcium and magnesium are excellent anti-allergy minerals that have a calming influence on the nervous system. They are found in nuts and seeds and green leafy vegetables. Prepare children who suffer from hay fever enticing salads full of green leafy vegetables and offer almonds as a snack if they are over five years old.

It is, as ever, important to encourage your child to drink plenty of fluids throughout the hay fever season. Water and diluted fresh juices help to thin mucus secretions.

Some naturopaths swear that the severity of hay fever symptoms can be reduced by taking a teaspoon of locally produced honey (made from local pollen) dissolved in warm water once a day in the run up to the hay fever season. The theory is that your child will gradually build up a resistance to the pollen that might cause full-blown symptoms once the hay fever season gets underway.

SUGGESTED RECIPES FOR HAY FEVER

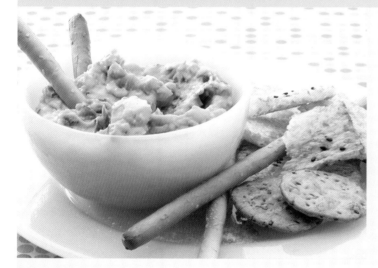

hay fever tonic

makes 2 large glasses or 4 small ones

This recipe requires an electric juicer. These are now available, reasonably priced, from many household shops.

½ cup (75 g/3 oz) blueberries
1 small cantaloupe melon, peeled
2 kiwi fruit, peeled
1 lemon, peeled with some pith left on
1 mango, peeled

Juice all of the above and drink straight away.

fresh lemonade

This is a delicious weekend treat for all the family as well as a therapeutic tonic for hay fever sufferers.

Juice and pulp of 8 lemons
1 cup (225 g/8 oz) fructose (fruit sugar)
A handful of ice cubes
1 pint sparkling or still water

Juice the lemons first. Put the lemon juice, fructose and ice cubes in a blender and liquidize to break up the ice and melt the fructose. Add the water slowly, mix well and serve immediately with straws.

guacamole

This recipe is packed full of the phytonutrient quercetin, vitamin C and beta-carotene, all of which may help ease hay fever symptoms.

2 ripe avocados, peeled and destoned
A small handful of coriander, chopped
2 garlic cloves, pressed
Juice of ½ a lemon
1 small red onion, finely chopped
2 ripe tomatoes, peeled and chopped
Sea salt and pepper to season

Lightly blend all the ingredients together in a food processor. Serve as a dip with corn crackers, rice cakes or grissini bread sticks.

headaches & migraines

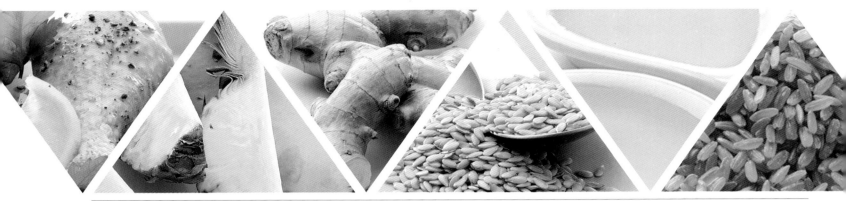

STAR FOODS FOR HEADACHES AND MIGRAINES: ALMOND, BLACKCURRANT, BROCCOLI, BROWN RICE, CAMOMILE, CARROT, CASHEW NUT, CHERRY, CHILLI PEPPER, EXTRA VIRGIN OLIVE OIL, FENNEL, GAME, GARLIC, GINGER, HONEY, KALE, LINSEED (FLAXSEED), MILLET, ONION, PARSLEY, PEAR, PINEAPPLE, ROCKET, WATERCRESS

There are many different causes of headaches. In children, they often occur through simple dehydration, especially after strenuous sporting activity. Encouraging your child to drink water regularly both at home and at school will prevent this from happening. Headaches can also be a symptom of stress. Anxiety can cause tension in the neck and shoulders, which constricts blood vessels to the head area causing pain. Eye strain is another common trigger than can lead to headaches. It is important to get a child's eyes tested if they suffer regularly. Other possible causes of headaches are poor posture, excessive caffeine intake, caffeine withdrawal, sinusitis, grinding teeth, injury or food allergies.

Migraines are severe headaches that occur on a regular basis and render the sufferer incapacitated for anything from several hours to several days. They are caused by the constriction and dilation of blood vessels around the brain and are frequently accompanied by nausea, dizziness and vomiting. The symptoms of migraine usually start in childhood or adolescence but they do not often manifest themselves as a headache. They are more likely to be in the form of dizziness, stomach pains, nausea, vomiting and severe motion sickness.

If your child were to get a sudden headache, accompanied by symptoms including a stiff neck, nausea, fever, sensitivity to bright lights and a rash, they could be suffering from meningitis or encephalitis and medical help must be sought immediately.

Treating headaches and migraine

Everyday headaches that are caused by stress, tension or dehydration respond well to fluid intake and rest. Using a blend of lavender and camomile oils in the bath can both soothe and comfort a child. Sleep is another wonderfully easy remedy for a headache. Persistent headaches, however, should be investigated because they can be a symptom of a more serious illness.

If your child or teenager suffers from migraine or migraine-type symptoms, it is imperative that they eat regularly. This helps to balance their blood sugar levels thereby avoiding hypoglycaemia, which appears to be a common symptom in migraine sufferers. Hypoglycaemia is low blood sugar. It occurs two to five hours after eating and is usually caused by an inadequate diet full of sugary foods, stimulants (such as caffeine) and refined foods. Symptoms of hypoglycaemia are fatigue, lightheadedness, dizziness, irritability, anxiety, cravings for sweet foods and an inability to concentrate.

Migraine is classed as an allergic condition. It often runs in families, especially where there is a history of other allergic conditions such as eczema, asthma or hay fever. Between 80 and 90 per cent of those affected by migraine suffer allergies or intolerances to some degree. For this reason, it is important to establish whether your child's migraines are triggered by any food or combination of foods. The most straightforward way to do this is for your child to undergo an exclusion diet (see right).

Studies have shown that the blood platelets of migraine sufferers clump and stick together more than usual and that this may lead to the onset of an attack. Eating foods containing nutrients that prevent platelet stickiness may be effective in some cases. (Of course, avoid any foods that are on an exclusion list if following a migraine exclusion diet.) These nutrients are vitamins B6, C, E and essential fatty acids (EFAs). Foods rich in vitamins B6 and E include peppers, green leafy vegetables, and nuts and seeds and their oils. Citrus fruits, blackcurrants and peppers are good sources of vitamin C. EFAs are found in evening primrose oil and linseed oil. Ginger is also known for its anti-platelet aggregatory effects.

The migraine exclusion diet

This diet excludes the major foods associated with migraine. It should be conducted under the guidance of a nutritionist who can assist with diet sheets and menu plans. Follow the guidelines and avoid the foods listed for one month.

• Any foods containing caffeine. This includes coffee, tea, chocolate, cocoa and fizzy drinks containing caffeine such as cola and "high energy" drinks.

• Any refined sugar that may upset your child's blood sugar levels. This means avoiding sweets, biscuits, pastries, cakes, as well as soft drinks that may contain sugar.

• Foods containing histamine: cheese, tuna, sardines, anchovies, salami, sausages, sauerkraut, spinach and tomato ketchup.

• Foods containing tyramine: cheese, chocolate, yeast extract, orange juice, tomato juice, fish and meats that are pickled, canned or smoked, nuts and seeds (except cashew nuts and linseeds), raspberries, red plums, avocados, bananas, potatoes and preserved pork products such as ham, bacon and sausages

• Food additives: tartrazine (E102), benzoate (E210–219), butylated hydroxytolueune (E321) and monosodium glutamate (E621)

• Wheat and dairy products

After the exclusion period, if your child has improved, you can reintroduce foods one at a time with a 3–7 day interval between each food. This will help to establish which foods are helpful and which are not. If your child does not improve during the course of the exclusion, then a more restricted diet can be used. This needs to be conducted under medical supervision. If you can distinguish the foods to which your child is reacting, eliminate them for a further three months and retest. After this time you may find that you can include the allergic foods in your child's diet again on a rotation basis (offering that food once every four days). However, some children may have to continue to avoid the culprit foods altogether.

SUGGESTED RECIPES FOR HEADACHES

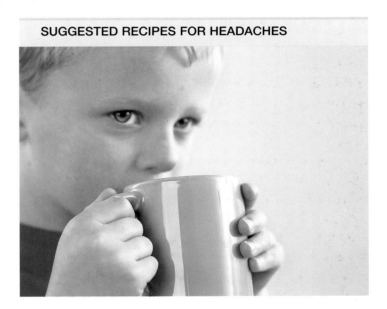

camomile and honey tea

serves one

A handful of camomile flowers
Boiling water
1 tsp honey

Put the camomile flowers in a teapot, cover with water and allow to steep for 5 minutes. Pour into a mug and stir in the honey.

ginger tea

serves one

1 slice ginger, crushed
1 tsp honey
Boiling water

Place the ginger in a mug, add the honey and pour over the boiling water. Allow the tea to cool slightly and sip slowly.

measles

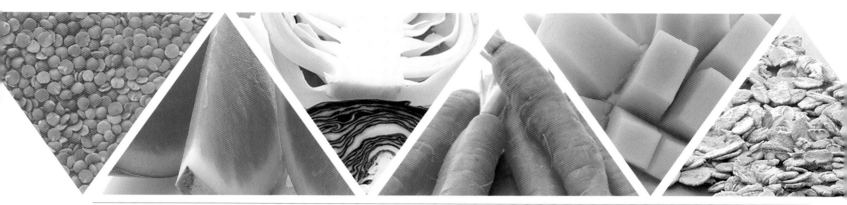

STAR FOODS FOR MEASLES: APPLE, APRICOT, BARLEY, BROCCOLI, BROWN RICE, CABBAGE, CANTALOUPE MELON, CARROT, CHICKPEA, KALE, KIWI FRUIT, LENTILS, MANGO, OATS, ORANGE, POULTRY, PRAWN, PUMPKIN AND PUMPKIN SEED, SUNFLOWER SEED, SWEET POTATO, SQUASH, WATERMELON

Measles is a highly contagious air-borne viral infection that passes from one child to another through coughing and sneezing. Children are currently vaccinated against measles at around 15 months old, often along with rubella and mumps. This combined vaccination is known as the MMR and is highly controversial due to the feared link with autism and a bowel disorder. As a result, some parents have chosen not to give their children the vaccination and, in places, take up is at an all-time low. Health authorities warn that a measles epidemic could occur if children are not vaccinated against this childhood disease. Vaccinations are not always 100 per cent effective, however, and regardless of whether or not you have vaccinated your child against measles, it is important to know how to protect them from the virus and how to help boost their defences should they contract it.

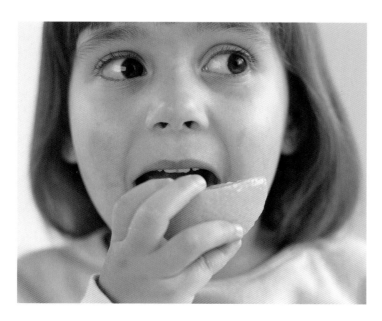

Measles begins with a cold and cough, fever, sore and itchy eyes and the appearance of small red spots with a white centre on the inside of the mouth. These are called Koplik's spots and are the symptom that differentiates measles from a general viral infection. Three to five days later the measles rash appears. It is browny-pink in colour and starts around the ears, face and neck before spreading to the rest of the body. It is usually only mildly itchy and lasts for four to seven days before fading away. Complications that can arise from measles include ear infections, pneumonia, eye problems and, in rare cases, encephalitis. A child with measles will feel very ill. They should be kept in bed and will often be more comfortable in a dimly lit room as their eyes may become sensitive to bright lights.

Medicinal foods for measles

Although a special diet won't be able to cure measles, certain important nutrients can have a huge impact on the disease. Measles depletes the stores of vitamin A in your child's body. Vitamin A is a fat-soluble vitamin that is stored in the liver. Deficiency symptoms of vitamin A include poor night vision and inflammation of the eyes, frequent colds and infections, mouth ulcers, dry skin, diarrhoea and dandruff. Research in developing countries, where nutrition is often poor and measles is still a serious killer, has shown that many deaths from measles could be prevented by administering a simple vitamin A supplement. Death from measles is extremely rare in developed, well-nourished countries but diet still has a crucial role to play in not only the prevention but also the treatment of this disease.

Vitamin A is found in both plant- and animal-based foods. The animal form of vitamin A, retinol, is found in abundance in full-fat dairy products, eggs, oily fish and liver. However, none of these foods are ideal to give to a sick child. Moreover, she simply will not feel like eating any of the above while she is ill. The best way to boost your child's intake of vitamin A is to offer her foods and drinks that are rich in the plant-based form of vitamin A, beta-carotene. Beta-carotene is converted into vitamin A by your child's body as and when it needs it. It is found in brightly coloured fruits and vegetables, such as apricot, carrot, squash, pumpkin, cantaloupe melon, watermelon, sweet potato, mango, broccoli, cabbage, kale and other green leafy vegetables.

Beta-carotene is also an antioxidant, which means that it helps to boost your child's immune system generally by fighting the harmful free radicals that cause disease. This is especially important when the body is under attack from a strong viral infection such as measles. Foods rich in beta-carotene are often also rich in vitamin C, another important antioxidant vitamin that will help your child to fight the infection. Good vitamin C sources are citrus fruits, peppers, berries, blackcurrants, parsley, broccoli, papaya, mango and apple.

Zinc is another nutrient with a role to play in both the prevention and treatment of this disease. It helps to mobilize stores of vitamin A from the liver as well as supporting the growth and development of white blood cells, the immune-army stalwarts that help protect your child from infection. You can now get suckable zinc lozenges for children from health food shops. Foods rich in zinc include shellfish, poultry, game, lean red meat, pulses, seeds, nuts and wholegrains.

While your child is in the initial stages of measles, offer her diluted fresh fruit and vegetable juices. Remember that children with a fever can become rapidly dehydrated, so it is important to provide plenty of enticing fluids. Homemade fruit juice ice pops can be comforting, as can vitamin- and mineral-packed soups and broths. Avoid sugary, fatty foods that impede the healing process, and dairy products, which may increase the risk of developing ear infections. As they feel better, introduce some vitamin A-rich foods, such as boiled eggs with wholemeal toast soldiers and diluted fresh orange juice.

SUGGESTED RECIPES FOR MEASLES

apple and carrot tonic

makes one glass

Packed with beta-carotene and vitamin C, this is a good tonic for children with measles.

2 eating apples, peeled and cored
1 carrot, peeled
Filtered or bottled water

Chop the apples and carrot into four. Feed through a juicer and dilute 50:50 with water.

immunity soup

This vegetable soup is full of immune-boosting vitamins and herbs. It is light and easy to digest. As your child gets better you can add some cooked chicken or chickpeas for a more filling meal.

1 medium onion, chopped
1 garlic clove, crushed
1 tbsp extra virgin olive oil
½ butternut squash, peeled and cubed
1 carrot, peeled and cubed
1 slice ginger
A handful of pot barley
1 sweet potato, cubed
1 sprig of thyme
850 ml (1½ pints) vegetable stock
1 head of broccoli
A handful of fresh parsley

Cook the onion and the garlic in the olive oil until transparent. Add all of the other ingredients except the broccoli and parsley and stir well. Cover and simmer for 30 minutes. Add the broccoli and simmer for a further 5 minutes. Sprinkle the parsley over the soup before serving. If your child does not like lumpy soup you can liquidize it for a smooth texture.

sore throats

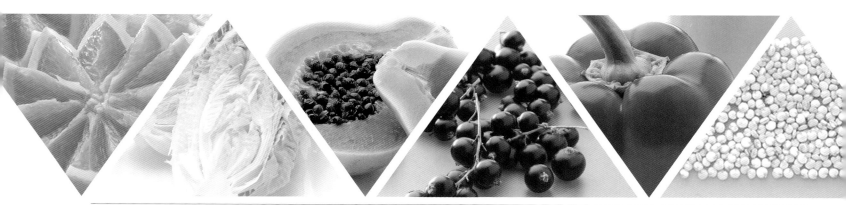

STAR FOODS FOR SORE THROATS: APRICOT, BARLEY, BLACKCURRANT, BOK CHOI, BROCCOLI, BROWN RICE, CARROT, CHICKEN, GARLIC, KALE, LEMON, LETTUCE, LIME, MANGO, MILLET, ONION, ORANGE, PAPAYA, QUINOA, RED PEPPER, SQUASH, SWEET POTATO, TURKEY, WATERCRESS

Sore throats are among the most common of childhood complaints. The symptoms are a raw, scratchy or burning sensation at the back of the throat that feels worse when swallowing. In childhood, sore throats are most often caused by viral infections such as the common cold. However, some sore throats are caused by bacterial infection, as in the case of streptococcus, often referred to as "strep throat". This is more common in children over three years of age and there are distinct differences between the symptoms of strep throat and those of a viral sore throat. Strep throat can come on very fast; one minute your child will be fine and the next they will have a very sore throat that may be accompanied by a headache, vomiting and a fever of up to 40°C (104°F). A viral sore throat usually appears gradually and is not necessarily accompanied by a fever. With strep throat, the tonsils will look swollen and red with white blotches on them and your child will look and feel really unwell.

Sore throats can also be caused by environmental factors such as dust, smoke and fumes. Persistent sore throats can be a symptom of another childhood disease or condition such as flu, chicken pox, measles, oral thrush, tonsillitis, glandular fever or chronic fatigue syndrome.

Tonsillitis is an acute sore throat, which is caused by the inflammation of the tonsils that sit on the left and right side of your child's throat. It can be either viral or bacterial and is more common in childhood than adulthood. Symptoms are similar to those of the sore throat but are far more acute and are often accompanied by a fever. Some children get recurrent tonsillitis and in rare cases this may lead to a tonsillectomy (an operation to remove the tonsils). This used to be a routine operation that was recommended to many children, along with the removal of the adenoids. Today, however, doctors realise the importance of the tonsils for the proper functioning of the immune system. Tonsils are important lymphoid tissue. This means that they contain white blood cells that help to fight a throat infection or an allergic reaction. Tonsils are now never removed unless absolutely necessary.

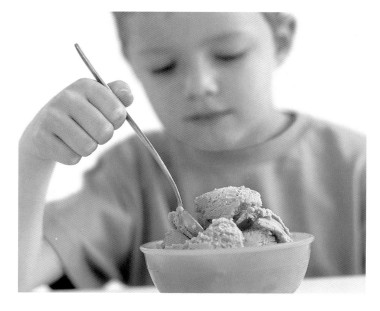

Medicinal foods for sore throats

A child with a sore throat, whether from a viral or bacterial infection, is unlikely to want to eat very much, partly because of the physical discomfort caused by swallowing. Offer plenty of water and fresh diluted fruit juices to support the lymphatic system and help ease her discomfort. If the child has a fever, adequate fluid intake is essential to prevent dehydration. Choose fruits and fruit juices rich in vitamin C, which has antiviral, antibacterial, anti-inflammatory and antioxidant properties. Blackcurrants and citrus fruits are excellent sources of vitamin C. For an extra boost, blackcurrants also provide a good supply of anthocyanins, phytonutrients that help reduce the inflammation associated with sore throats and have antioxidant powers 20 times stronger than vitamin C and 50 times the strength of vitamin E. Antioxidants help the immune system to combat free radicals, the cell-altering, disease-causing atoms that the body is fighting constantly.

Foods rich in beta-carotene are also advisable to help soothe a sore throat. Beta-carotene has similar antioxidant and membrane-healing qualities to vitamin C and can be found in all brightly coloured fruits and vegetables. If your child is not very hungry, all of these can be juiced or added to soups. Garlic is a wonderful food for sore throats as it is antibacterial, antiviral and antifungal. Add it to soups, juices and dressings, or offer it as a syrup (see right).

During the acute phase of a sore throat, avoid dairy products, which tend to increase mucus production. Mucus is a breeding-ground for bacteria and any excess will leave your child feeling blocked up. Also reduce her intake of sugar and refined foods as these will suppress immune activity and may prolong the illness.

As your child's sore throat improves, encourage her to eat meals rich in wholegrains, lean meat, fish and plenty of fruits and vegetables. This will supply all the nutrients needed for the immune system to function efficiently.

If your child has to take antibiotics, wait until the course has finished and then offer live natural yoghurt every day for a month to replace the friendly bacteria in the gut that has been eliminated by the antibiotics. For children with dairy allergy, you can buy dairy-free probiotic powders from health food shops which can be added to drinks or dairy-free yoghurts.

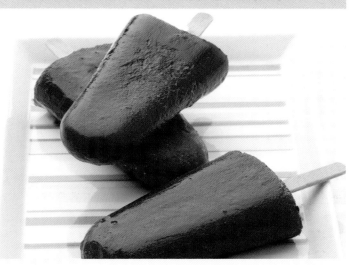

blackcurrant and strawberry ice pops

These delicious ice pops are rich in vitamin C to boost immune function and help to soothe the mucous membranes in the throat.

1 cup (115 g/4 oz) blackcurrants, destalked
1 cup (115 g/4 oz) strawberries
4 tbsp fructose
1 cup (225 g/8 oz) apple juice

In a liquidizer, whizz up all the ingredients until smooth. Sieve the mixture to remove the seeds and pour into lolly moulds. Freeze until they are set.

garlic and honey syrup

Garlic is renowned for its antibacterial and antiviral properties. Add Manuka honey, which is a natural antiseptic, to help chase away any unwanted bugs.

4 tbsp Manuka honey
2 garlic cloves, pressed

Place the honey and garlic in a bowl, cover and leave to soak for a few hours. Strain the mixture and place in a sealed glass container in the fridge. Give your child a teaspoon of syrup, 3 times a day. It will taste quite spicy and you can offer a chaser of undiluted fruit juice if necessary.

ear infections

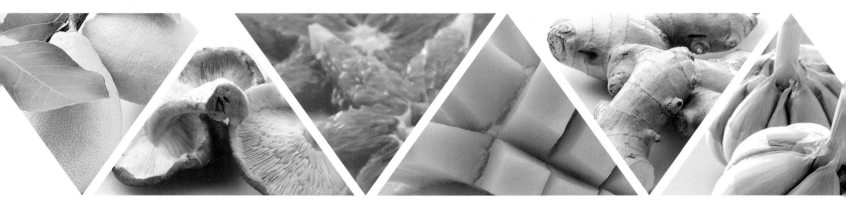

STAR FOODS FOR EAR INFECTIONS: BEETROOT, BLUEBERRY, CANTALOUPE MELON, CARROT, CELERY, CHICKEN, CHILLI, GARLIC, GINGER, GRAPEFRUIT, GUAVA, HORSERADISH, KIWI FRUIT, LEMON, LIME, MANGO, ONION, ORANGE, PARSLEY, PUMPKIN, SHIITAKE MUSHROOM, SWEET POTATO, TOFU

Ear infections are very common in childhood and are most prevalent between the ages of six months and three years. Children in this age group are more likely to develop ear infections because the part of the ear known as the Eustachian tube, which links the ear with the nose and throat, lies more horizontally in them than it does in older children. This causes drainage problems when fluid collects, encouraging the growth of bacteria. As children grow older, the Eustachian tube develops a curve that makes drainage much easier and lowers the risk of ear infections.

The symptoms of an ear infection are earache, a fever and a feeling of pressure in the ear. The pressure is caused by the build-up of fluid pushing against the ear drum. Babies with ear infections are often distressed and pull at the affected ear, which can turn bright red externally. Ear infections may occur during or after a cold or other respiratory illness.

Chronic ear infections can lead to permanent hearing damage, although this is not common. Always seek medical advice for an ear infection as, left untreated, it can cause perforation of the ear drum. Recurrent ear infections can result in glue ear. This is caused by a build-up of thick, sticky mucus behind the ear drum causing temporary, partial deafness. Ear infections are conventionally treated with antibiotics. However, repeated use of antibiotics brings its own problems and recent studies have found that children routinely treated with these drugs were far more likely to get

SUGGESTED RECIPES FOR EAR INFECTIONS

immune-boosting chicken broth

1 chicken
2 medium onions, cut into quarters
4 garlic cloves
1 tbsp fresh ginger, chopped
1 red chilli, deseeded
4 large carrots, chopped
4 sticks celery, chopped
2 litres (2½ pints) vegetable stock
1 cup (150 g/5½ oz) fresh peas
1 cup (90 g/3 oz) broccoli florets
A large handful of coriander and parsley, chopped
Juice of 2 limes

Place the chicken, onion, garlic, ginger, chilli, carrots and celery into a large pan. Cover with the stock, bring to the boil and simmer with the lid on for 1 hour, or until the chicken is cooked through and beginning to fall off the bone. Remove the chicken from the pan and separate the meat from the skin and bones, which can be discarded. Strain the remaining liquid or broth through a colander and skim off any excess fat. Return the chicken and broth back to the pan and add the peas and broccoli. Simmer for 10 minutes until the vegetables are cooked through. Add the coriander, parsley and lime juice and serve immediately. For young children you can liquidize the broth to form a smooth soup. Portions of this soup can also be frozen to use when needed.

recurrent ear infections than those who managed to avoid using them. For parents, the decision of whether or not to give a child antibiotics can be hard and one of the roles of nutrition in addressing childhood illness is to help avert the need for such a dilemma.

Medicinal foods for ear infections

Breastfed babies are less likely to suffer from ear infections than bottle-fed babies because they employ a greater sucking action, which helps the ear to stay clear of mucus. Breast milk also contains plenty of antimicrobial substances to protect your baby. If you are bottle-feeding your baby, be sure to feed in an upright rather than a flat position. This will prevent fluid and air from entering the Eustachian tube where a bacterial infection could easily develop.

Avoid smoking around a baby or young child. There is a direct link between smoky environments and ear infections in children. In 80 per cent of children tested in one study, recurrent ear infections cleared up once smoke was eliminated from their environment.

If your child does show the symptoms of an ear infection, act fast. Make some ear drops by crushing a clove of garlic and covering it with ½ cup (115 ml/4 fl oz) extra virgin olive oil. Mix well and leave for 15 minutes. After this time, take a teaspoon of the oil (not containing any of the garlic pieces) and gently heat over a low flame. Allow it to cool slightly and then transfer to a dropper (available from chemists). Lay your child on her side and place one or two drops of warm, not hot, oil into the ear. This can soothe any pain and garlic, which is antibacterial, can help to heal the infection.

Children with recurrent ear infections should be tested for food allergies as these have been implicated as an underlying cause of infection in some cases. Dairy products are the most common culprit. Other possibilities are wheat, corn, egg, peanuts, peanut butter and citrus fruits. If your child has an ear infection they should avoid dairy products anyway because these thicken and increase mucus, making it more difficult for an infected ear to drain. This includes milk, cream, ice cream, cheese and yoghurt. Replace these foods with other sources of calcium, minerals and protein – such as nuts and seeds, beans, fortified rice drinks and soya products, molasses and green leafy vegetables. Other foods that increase mucus include egg, red meat, fried foods and those containing sugar or salt.

Foods that help to break down mucus include citrus fruits, garlic, onion, celery, parsley, chicken broth, chilli, watercress, horseradish and green tea. Offer your child a hot toddy of lemon and honey and prepare an immune-boosting chicken broth (left) to aid the healing process. Make fresh juices from antioxidant-rich fruits and vegetables, such as orange, mango, papaya, cantaloupe melon, kiwi fruit, blackcurrants, blueberries and carrot to help your child fight the infection.

If your child has to take antibiotics, wait until the course has finished and then offer live yoghurt every day for a month to replace the friendly bacteria eliminated from her gut. For children with a dairy allergy, you can buy dairy-free probiotic powders from health food shops, which can be added to drinks or dairy-free yoghurts.

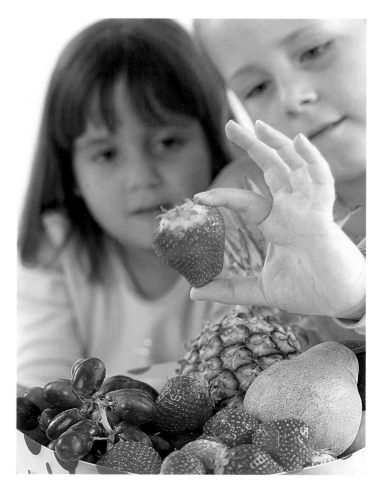

cancer

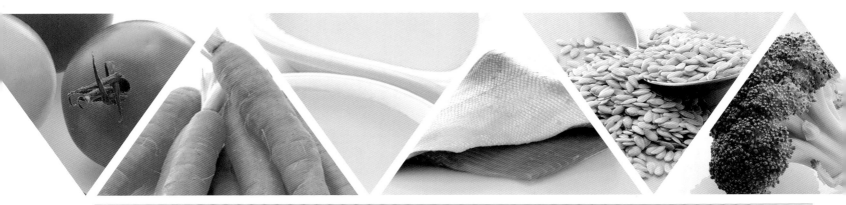

STAR FOODS FOR CANCER: ALFAFA SPROUT, ALMOND, APPLE, APRICOT, ASPARAGUS, BEANS, BEANSPROUT, BRAZIL NUT, BROCCOLI, BROWN RICE, BRUSSELS SPROUT, CARROT, CAULIFLOWER, CHICORY, EVENING PRIMROSE OIL, EXTRA VIRGIN OLIVE OIL, GARLIC, GINGER, GREEN TEA, KALE, LENTILS, LETTUCE, LINSEED AND LINSEED OIL, MANGO, PEA, PULSES, PUMPKIN SEED, QUINOA, SALMON, SESAME SEED, SHIITAKE MUSHROOM, SOYA MILK, SUNFLOWER SEED, SWEET POTATO, TOFU, TOMATO, TURMERIC

Cancer kills more children than any other disease in the developed world. In the US, one in every 330 children develops some form of the disease before the age of 20. In European countries, it is estimated that one out of every 500 children will be diagnosed with cancer before they reach the age of 15.

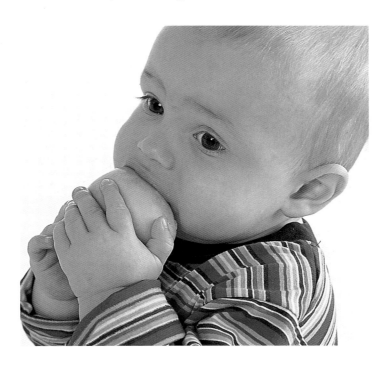

Cancer occurs when ordinary healthy cells in the body mutate and multiply. When a cell is damaged (by free radicals, for example) it develops abnormally and then divides and multiplies in its damaged form. A build-up of these cancerous cells creates a tumour. This process of cell damage is happening all the time in our bodies and, usually, antioxidants in the body keep this process in check. Cancer forms when the body's protective mechanisms are overwhelmed. Cancer cells divide and multiply uncontrollably. They also have the ability to metastasize, meaning that they spread through the lymphatic system and bloodstream and appear in other parts of the body.

Childhood and adult cancers differ. When first diagnosed, children generally have an advanced form of their particular cancer. In 80 per cent of cases, it will already have spread to distant sites. With adult cancers, two thirds are caused by smoking and poor diet and less than 20 per cent will already have spread on diagnosis. One reason for the far higher rate of metastasis in childhood cancers may be that childhood is a time of great growth, and this includes both healthy and unhealthy development. The most commonly diagnosed types of childhood cancer are leukaemia and cancer of the brain or the lymphatic system. Less common are cancers of the bone, muscles, kidneys and nervous system. While childhood cancer is often at a relatively advanced stage when diagnosed, the good news is that up to 70 per cent of children with the disease can now be cured.

Medicinal foods for cancer

The main aim of this section is to provide dietary information on supporting a child during and after treatment for cancer. Such a child will need feeding with great care and attention to build them back up to a healthy state of being and there are certain foods that are known to be anticarcinogenic that can help with this process.

Children undergoing chemotherapy are likely to lose their appetite and suffer dramatic weight loss. Frequent small meals and snacks high in vegetable protein, soluble fibre and essential fatty acids will help to redress the balance. Children on hormone therapy (steroids) often develop insatiable appetites and gain weight rapidly. They also have a tendency to retain water, which further adds to their weight gain. For these children, a diet high in fruit and vegetables, which will help to eradicate the excess water, is recommended. They should also avoid fatty foods and instead eat wholegrains with fish and sources of vegetable protein, such as soya products, beans, pulses, nuts and seeds. Snacks should consist of fruit, vegetables with dips and corn crackers, muesli bars, muffins and cakes.

In general terms, serve a child with cancer a diet rich in wholegrains such as brown rice, wholemeal bread and pasta, millet, oats, barley, rye and quinoa. The fibre these foods contain helps to balance blood glucose levels and to carry toxins and carcinogens out of the body. Include plenty of cruciferous vegetables, such as broccoli, in the diet as these contain anticarcinogenic compounds. Offer lots of colourful fruits and vegetables (red, yellow, orange, blue and black) and juice them to provide concentrated forms of their high levels of vitamins and phytonutrients. Vitamin C-rich foods have a restorative effect partly because vitamin C is used to make collagen, which strengthens cell membranes, thereby helping to stop the cancer cells from multiplying. Other key anticarcinogens are onion and garlic. Add them to soups, broths and juices. Almonds contain a substance called laetrile, which has anti-cancer properties. They can be served raw as a snack or as almond milk (see page 113).

Avoid dairy products and high-fat meat products. Cancer thrives on arachidonic acid, which is a by-product of fat metabolism. Also, chemotherapy sometimes causes lactose intolerance in children. Protein should come mainly from vegetable sources such as soya products, beans, pulses, grains, nuts and seeds as well as fish if well tolerated. Also avoid refined sugar, flour, processed and refined foods and salt, all of which suppress immune function and can cause blood sugar fluctuations.

Nutritional supplements are usually advised in addition to a good diet. However, always seek guidance from a nutritionist specializing in cancer before giving your child any vitamins or minerals.

SUGGESTED RECIPES FOR CANCER

protein shake
serves one

For children feeling very weak and nauseous, protein drinks can be enormously beneficial. This recipe is liquid food full of protein, vitamins and essential fats.

1 cup (225 ml/8 fl oz) apple juice
1 ripe banana
1 tsp brewer's yeast
1 tbsp linseed (flaxseed) oil
¼ cup (60 ml/2 fl oz) silken tofu
½ cup (60 g/2 oz) strawberries (or any other fruit)

In a liquidizer, blend all the ingredients together and serve through a straw. Add more apple juice if too thick for your child's liking.

carrot, orange and ginger booster juice
serves one

You need an electric juicer for this recipe. This juice is an excellent way of giving your child high levels of the carotenoids that many studies have shown to be anticarcinogenic. The ginger might help with any nausea that accompanies treatment.

1 slice fresh ginger
2 large carrots
2 oranges

Juice the ginger first, followed by the carrots and oranges. Serve straight away.

diabetes

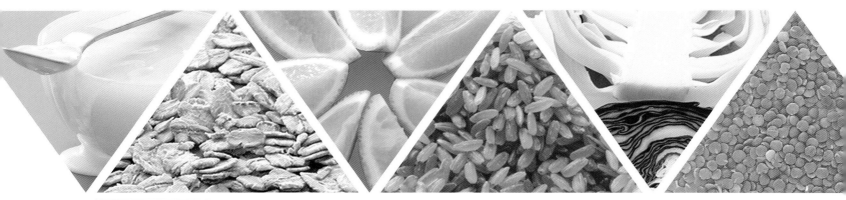

STAR FOODS FOR DIABETES: ALMOND, APPLE, BAKED BEAN, BERRIES, BROCCOLI, BROWN RICE, BUTTER BEAN, CABBAGE, CASHEW NUT, CAULIFLOWER, CHICKPEA, EGG YOLK, FRUCTOSE, GARLIC, KALE, KIDNEY BEAN, LENTILS, LETTUCE, LOW-FAT NATURAL YOGHURT, OAT BRAN, OATS, ORANGE, PEANUT, PEAR, PUMPKIN SEED, RYE BREAD, RYE CRACKER, SEAFOOD, SESAME SEED, SOYA BEAN, SPIRULINA, SUNFLOWER SEED, WHOLEMEAL BREAD, WHOLEMEAL PASTA

Diabetes affects around one in 50 people in the UK and as many as one in 20 in the US. It is a chronic condition caused by a deficiency of the hormone insulin, which is produced by the pancreas. Insulin plays an important role in metabolism and blood sugar balance in the body. Once your child has eaten, her body gets busy breaking down the food, digesting it and converting it into glucose, which the body can then use to refuel its cells. When the glucose has entered the bloodstream for transportation, insulin controls the amount of glucose in the blood and the rate at which it is absorbed by cells. It acts like a key to the cells: without insulin, the glucose cannot enter the cells at all and the body cannot function. If your child has diabetes, there is a lack of insulin in the body that causes glucose to build up in the blood instead of being delivered to the cells. This leads to hyperglycaemia (high blood sugar levels), which is a dangerous condition that can lead to many complications including kidney disease, heart disease, eye disorders and nerve damage. Symptoms of diabetes include frequent urinating, frequent infections, unquenchable thirst, weight loss, fatigue, mood swings and irritability. In children, excessive bed-wetting can be another symptom.

There are two types of diabetes. Type I diabetes, also called insulin-dependant diabetes mellitus (IDDM) or juvenile onset diabetes, usually starts at an early age and is considered to be an autoimmune disorder. For reasons not yet known, the body's immune system attacks and destroys the insulin-producing cells in the pancreas. Some experts believe that a genetic predisposition to diabetes along with an exposure to a viral infection may trigger the onset of the disease. In addition, there is some evidence that allergy to bovine serum albumin (BSA), a blood protein found in dairy products, may play a part and that this may cause the child's

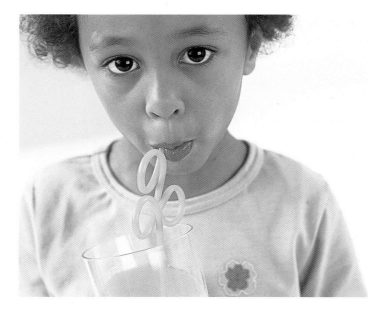

immune system to malfunction and attack the cells of the pancreas. Children and adults with this type of diabetes have to inject daily with insulin and monitor their blood glucose levels carefully.

Type II diabetes, which is also called non-insulin-dependant diabetes mellitus, is more common than Type I. This type of diabetes usually occurs later in life and is associated with obesity. However, obesity is becoming a major problem in children in the developed world and recent research has revealed that increasing numbers of young children are showing the early warning signs of a developing resistance to insulin as a result of being overweight or obese. This insulin resistance is believed to be an early indicator of both types of diabetes but particularly Type II, in which the body produces some insulin but the body tissues have developed a resistance to it. Type II diabetes is controlled through diet and oral insulin tablets.

The diabetes diet

Controlling blood sugar levels is of paramount importance for sufferers of both Type I and Type II diabetes. Diabetics should never miss meals nor over-eat. Eating frequent small meals is the best way to avoid wild fluctuations in blood sugar levels. A child with diabetes, like other children, should eat three meals and two snacks a day. The diet should be low in fat and high in fibre with plenty of fruits and vegetables, wholegrains, beans and pulses. Fibre, especially oat bran, helps to reduce blood sugar surges. Diabetics are at a higher risk of heart disease and, as such, should avoid fatty foods such as full-fat dairy products, fatty cuts of meat, fat-laden snacks and fast food. Most protein should come from vegetable sources such as beans, pulses and grains.

Snacks should be made from fruit, wholegrain rye, oat or rice crackers with nut butters, raw vegetables and dips, and low-fat dairy products such as cottage cheese. Sweet and sugary foods along with refined foods such as white flour, white rice, white pasta and white sugar should be used sparingly and are best avoided.

Exercise also has an important part to play in diabetes control. Studies have shown that regular exercise increases insulin sensitivity and can therefore reduce the number of injections required. It also reduces cholesterol and tryglyceride (blood fat) levels and helps with weight loss in overweight diabetics.

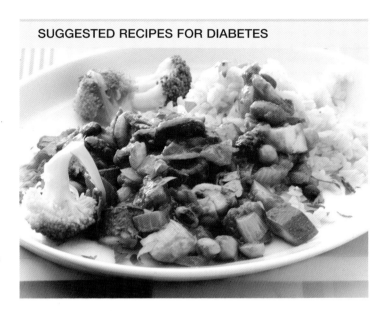

SUGGESTED RECIPES FOR DIABETES

mixed bean stew

This dish can help to stabilize blood sugar levels.

1 onion, chopped
1 tbsp extra virgin olive oil
1 handful of mushrooms, chopped
1 garlic clove, crushed
1 tin of chopped tomatoes (no-sugar, no-salt variety)
1 courgette, diced
1 tin of mixed pulses
A handful of flat leaf parsley, chopped

In a saucepan, sauté the onion in the olive oil until transparent. Add the mushrooms and garlic and cook for a couple of minutes. Add all of the rest of the ingredients except the parsley and gently simmer for 15 minutes until the vegetables are cooked. Sprinkle with the parsley and serve with brown rice and broccoli florets.

oatbran and berries smoothie

serves one

1 ripe banana
1 cup (225 ml/8 fl oz) calcium-enriched soya milk
A handful of ice cubes
1 tbsp oat bran
1 tbsp porridge oats
1 cup (115 g/4 oz) strawberries

Whizz all the ingredients together in a liquidizer. Serve immediately.

coeliac disease

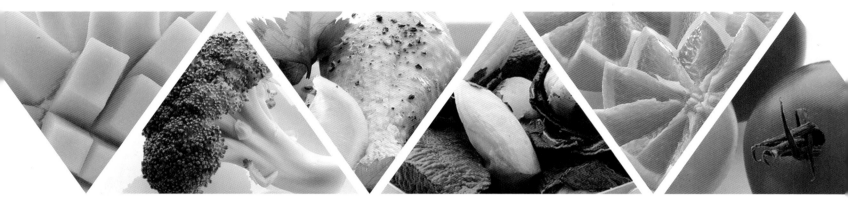

STAR FOODS FOR COELIAC DISEASE: ALMOND, AMARANTH, APPLE, APRICOT, BANANA, BEANS, BRAZIL NUT, BROCCOLI, BUCKWHEAT, CANTALOUPE MELON, CARROT, CASHEW NUT, CORN, DRIED APRICOT, GAME, LENTILS, LETTUCE, LINSEED, MANGO, MILLET, MOLASSES, PEAR, PEA, POTATO, POULTRY, PUMPKIN SEED, QUINOA, RAISIN, RASPBERRY, RICE, SEAFOOD, SESAME SEED, STRAWBERRY, SUNFLOWER SEED, SWEET POTATO, SWEETCORN, TOMATO, WATERMELON

Coeliac disease is a hereditary digestive disorder that affects about one in 1500 people in the UK and up to one in 500 in the US. It is caused by a sensitivity to gluten in certain grains. Gluten is the protein found in wheat, kamut, spelt, triticale, barley, oats and rye. Causal factors are unknown but it seems mostly to affect white Europeans or those of European descent and it does run in families.

Coeliac disease is often described as an autoimmune disease. This is because when a food containing gluten is consumed by the sufferer, the body recognizes it as an antigen, or foreign substance, and launches an immune assault. As a result, the lining of the small intestine, which is covered by small hair-like projections called villi, gets damaged and starts to atrophy. This leads to poor absorption of vital nutrients, resulting in malnutrition. Coeliac disease is a serious condition and if left untreated can be life-threatening.

A Dutch doctor during the Second World War first made the connection between gluten and the symptoms of coeliac disease. As a result of rationing and lack of flour (and therefore bread), most children were undernourished and thin. A small minority, however, appeared to thrive on the diet. These children had suffered from stomach illnesses before rationing began. Once the food situation improved these children fell ill again. The doctor experimented with their diet and discovered that wheat and rye were the cause of their problems. Later research identified the culprit as gluten.

Coeliac disease can first strike either in childhood or in adulthood. In children with a hereditary susceptibility, it usually occurs with the introduction of cereal products between four and eight months of age. In an infant, the symptoms are foul-smelling diarrhoea, failure to thrive, poor appetite and resulting lack of weight gain. With older children and adults the disease may be caused by emotional stress, a viral infection or a physical trauma such as surgery. The symptoms include abdominal pain and swelling, pale and foul-smelling diarrhoea, muscle cramps and aches, extreme tiredness and weight loss.

Coeliac disease is difficult to diagnose in children, as symptoms can be very similar to other common childhood disorders such as gastroenteritis, irritable bowel syndrome, food allergies or anaemia. Diagnosis is based on a blood test followed by an intestinal biopsy.

Another complication of coeliac disease can be an increased susceptibility to food allergies. This can occur as a result of the damage that the disease causes to the villi of the small intestine, making the intestine more permeable. A suspected food allergy (see pages 114–15) is quite a separate condition to coeliac disease but one that needs, equally, to be promptly addressed. The good news is that, if caught early, the damage to the intestines caused by coeliac disease does repair, as long as a gluten-free diet is adopted and maintained on a permanent basis.

The coeliac diet

Once diagnosed, children with coeliac disease will need to avoid gluten for the rest of their lives. This means avoiding any form of food made from wheat, rye, oats and barley, and triticale, kamut and spelt (old forms of wheat). This does not just mean avoiding bread, pasta and flour made from these grains. There are many hidden sources that also have to be eliminated to protect a coeliac child. It is important to learn to read food labels. Here are a few helpful hints:

- Avoid bread, pastas, flour, biscuits, cakes, crackers and pastry made from wheat
- Avoid rye breads, crackers, and pastas made from rye
- Avoid lemon barley water, malt and malt products, barley enzymes used to make rice milk and some brands of soya milk
- Avoid sauces and soups thickened with wheat flour
- Avoid food additives manufactured from the culprit grains such as caramel, MSG, maltose, malt, malt flavouring, gum base, citric acid, vegetable gum, maltodextrin and modified starch.
- Avoid hydrolyzed vegetable protein, textured vegetable protein, some soy sauces, beer, mustard, tomato ketchup, gravy powders, stock cubes, curry powder and seasonings

Oats contain a protein called avenin, which is similar to gluten. Recent studies have shown that people with coeliac disease may be able to tolerate avenin as it differs in structure from gluten. However, the oats must be grown, milled, packaged and transported away from wheat to avoid cross-contamination. Seek further advice from your doctor on this subject if any of your children are coeliacs.

Coeliacs need a diet high in non-gluten fibre, iron and B-vitamins. Good sources of fibre are fresh vegetables and fruit, beans, pulses and lentils, seeds and dried fruits. Molasses is an excellent source of iron as are game, poultry and dried fruits. Foods rich in B-vitamins include nuts and seeds, pulses, eggs, milk, fish, lean meat, dried fruits and green leafy vegetables. Also offer foods that contain high levels of beta-carotene and vitamin A, as these help to protect the mucous membranes in the small intestine. Foods that are a good source of beta-carotene include apricot, carrot, butternut squash, broccoli, sweet potato, spinach, watercress, cantaloupe melon, pumpkin, mango and papaya.

Some gluten-free recipes in this book include: watercress soup (page 63); coconut and cauliflower soup (page 63); seafood paella (page 66); millet porridge with date purée (page 72); chicken casserole (page 72); handy hummus with baked potato (page 74); venison shepherd's pie (page 74); baked apple with raisins and spices (page 75); parsley eggs (page 78); turkey and cranberry burgers (page 79); tuna fishcakes (page 79); pheasant paysanne (page 79); sweetcorn patties (page 81); strawberry smoothie (page 83); kiwi and banana smoothie (page 83); venison burgers (page 88); chicken and almond satay with carrot and sesame stir-fry (page 88); tuna and prawn brochette with coriander marinade (page 89); cod and parma ham parcels with red pesto (page 89); salmon lollipops (page 89); papaya and lime smoothie (page 91); rustic saturday soup (page 95); stir-fry duck strips with orange and ginger (page 97); family paella (page 98); queen scallop stir-fry (page 98).

SUGGESTED RECIPES FOR COELIAC DISEASE

gluten-free chocolate brownie birthday cake

serves 8

This is a once-a-year recipe that can be devoured by all the family. You would not even know that it was made with gluten-free flour. Use exact measurements for the best results.

100 g (3½ oz) unhydrogenated vegetable margarine (or butter if dairy-tolerant)
75 g (2¾ oz) 70% cocoa cooking chocolate
100 g (3½ oz) gluten-free flour (available in supermarkets)
1 tsp baking powder
100 g (3½ oz) finely chopped walnuts
175 g (6 oz) fructose (fruit sugar)
3 eggs, beaten

Preheat the oven to 180°C/350°F/Gas Mark 4. In a saucepan, melt together the butter and chocolate. In a separate bowl, mix together the flour, baking powder, nuts and fructose. Add the beaten eggs followed by the melted butter and chocolate. Pour into an oiled cake tin and bake in the oven for 45–50 minutes. The cake should remain sticky. Allow to cool in the tin and then transfer to a plate. As the cake is so sticky, you won't need to ice it.

other illnesses

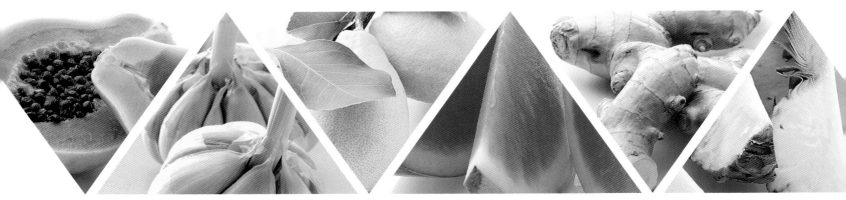

vomiting and diarrhoea

STAR FOODS: NO FOOD FOR 24–48 HOURS

Whether as a result of a viral or bacterial infection or food poisoning, both vomiting and diarrhoea can be serious for babies and young children as they can easily become dehydrated. A child of any age suffering from these illnesses should be kept hydrated by being offered plenty of water to drink. If your child is vomiting frequently, give her a rehydration drink. You can buy these in sachets from a chemist or you can make your own (see opposite). Make sure that your child sips any drink slowly as sometimes even liquid can precipitate another bout of vomiting. Diarrhoea often accompanies vomiting. It is characterized by frequent, watery stools and is the body's way of eliminating an unwanted substance or microbe from your child's gut.

If your child is sick and/or gets diarrhoea, avoid all food for 24 hours. Be especially careful to avoid all dairy products, including milk or formula, which will exacerbate the problem as diarrhoea can cause a temporary lactose intolerance. This does not apply to babies who are being exclusively breastfed because their mother's milk does not count as a dairy product. They should be protected from these conditions by antibodies and healthy bacteria present in breast milk anyway. For formula-fed babies, rice milk (available in supermarkets and health food shops) has traditionally been used to treat infant diarrhoea.

Once the vomiting and diarrhoea have abated, introduce foods that will be comforting to your child's digestive system and will help bring them back to full strength. Carrots and apples are traditional remedies for diarrhoea. Rice cakes and white rice act as a kind of nutritional blotting paper and will not irritate the sensitive mucous membranes of your child's digestive tract. Bananas are another good choice of food and will help to replace any potassium lost during the illness. They will also boost your child's energy levels after a bout of feeling weak. Soups and broths are comforting to eat and offer an easy way to help replace vitamins and minerals lost as a result of the illness.

If the diarrhoea or vomiting persists for more than a couple of days, consult your doctor as they may be a symptom of another illness or of a parasitic infection.

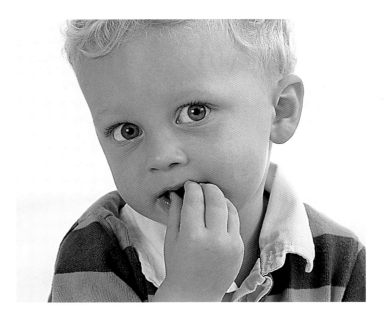

colds

STAR FOODS: BLACKCURRANT, CARROT, CHICKEN, CHILLI, GARLIC, GINGER, GUAVA, HORSERADISH, LEMON, LIME, ONION, ORANGE, PARSLEY, PEA, SQUASH, SWEET POTATO

There are more than 200 known viruses that cause colds. This number is ever-growing as viruses are constantly mutating to create new strains that the body does not recognize. On average, children suffer from between six and ten colds a year, whereas adults suffer from between two and four colds over the same period. How your child's body deals with a cold or, indeed, any viral infection, will be determined by the strength of her immune system and the foods that she eats during the course of the infection.

A diet rich in fruits and vegetables, wholegrains, nuts and seeds, pulses, lean meats and fish will strengthen your child's immune defences. Immune-boosting chicken broth (see page 126) helps to clear congestion and contains drug-like compounds very similar to the ones found in over-the-counter cold remedies.

Vitamin C and zinc have both been proved to reduce the severity and length of a cold. This is likely to be because vitamin C promotes the production of interferon – the body's natural antiviral agent. Zinc, particularly taken as a lozenge (available at chemists) seems to be highly effective at reducing the length of a cold as it appears to prevent the cold viruses from replicating.

fever

STAR FOODS: BLUEBERRY, CAMOMILE, CARROT, ECHINACEA, GARLIC, GINGER, GOLDEN SEAL, GRAPEFRUIT, LEMON, LIME, ORANGE, OREGANO, PAPAYA, PINEAPPLE, SAGE, THYME, WATERMELON

The normal temperature of a child is considered to be 37°C (98.6°F) if taken orally. If your child's temperature registers higher than this, she is considered to be feverish. A fever is not so much an illness but a signal that the body is trying to fight off something that shouldn't be there and is assisting the healing process through a natural means. Its cause is usually a bacterial or viral infection. The fever is caused by a chemical reaction that takes place while the immune army tries to destroy the invader. This causes the release of chemicals called pyrogens, which raise your child's body temperature. This helps the immune army in several ways. At a raised temperature your child's body produces more white blood cells, and her heart beats faster, making the blood pump around the body more quickly. This means that the white blood cells can travel to the site of infection faster. The heat produced by the fever also increases antibody production and interferon activity.

While a fever is present, do not encourage your child to eat sweet and fatty foods. Eating requires digestion and this takes up a great deal of energy that should be directed toward the healing process. Offer plenty of fluids, including water, diluted fruit juices, soups and broths, to prevent dehydration. This is very important as a feverish child will lose body fluids quickly.

Childhood fevers usually resolve themselves fairly rapidly. Only if a temperature appears to be spiralling out of control do you need worry. Never hesitate to seek medical help in cases of high fever or, indeed, if you are worried about your child's condition. If a fever is accompanied by a headache, sensitivity to bright lights, body rashes and a sore, stiff neck then consult your doctor immediately as these can be symptoms of meningitis, which is a medical emergency.

SUGGESTED RECIPES

anti-viral booster

serves one

1 banana
1 kiwi fruit
Juice of 4 oranges
A few drops of echinacea (age-dependant dosage)
A pinch of vitamin C powder

Whizz all the ingredients together in a liquidizer. Serve immediately.

rehydration drink

serves one

1 tsp sea salt
2 dessertspoons sugar
1 litre (1¾ pints) water
600 ml (1 pint) fresh orange juice

Mix together all of the ingredients. Offer one glass every hour after a bout of vomiting.

glossary

ALLERGEN a substance that causes an allergy.

AMINO ACID one of 20 basic building blocks of **protein**. All proteins in the body are made of a combination of two or more amino acids.

ANALGESIC a substance that relieves pain.

ANAPHYLACTIC SHOCK a severe form of allergic reaction in which the body releases vast quantities of **histamine** into the body, causing swelling and breathing difficulties. This is a medical emergency that requires immediate treatment.

ANTIBIOTIC a treatment for fungal or bacterial infections that works by killing, or inhibiting the growth of, the infecting organisms.

ANTIBODY a blood **protein** that can destroy bacteria and other harmful substances. Each antibody combats a particular infection. The body becomes immune to the infection once it has developed an effective antibody to it.

ANTICARCINOGENIC a substance that may inhibit the production of cancer in living cells.

ANTIHISTAMINE a substance that counteracts the effects of the **histamine** produced by the body in allergic reactions.

ANTI-INFLAMMATORY a substance that reduces inflammation.

ANTIOXIDANT a substance that inhibits and controls **free radicals**. Vitamins A, C and E, the minerals selenium and zinc, and many **phytonutrients** are important antioxidants.

ANTIVIRAL a substance that is effective in combating viruses.

AUTOIMMUNE DISEASE a condition whereby the body loses the ability to distinguish between "self" and foreign invaders and launches an immune assault against itself.

BACTERIA simple micro-organisms, some of which naturally occur in the human gut and are important in fighting infection (often called "friendly" bacteria), and some of which can be harmful and cause disease.

BETA-CAROTENE an **antioxidant** that can protect the body against **free radicals**. The body turns it into vitamin A as and when needed. Its pigmentation gives foods such as carrots and red peppers their bright colours.

CARCINOGEN a substance that may produce cancer in living cells.

COELIAC DISEASE a condition caused by sensitivity to **gluten**, a **protein** found in certain grains: wheat, oats, barley and rye. These foods damage the small intestine, leading to poor absorption of vital nutrients. As a result, the sufferer needs to follow a gluten-free diet.

COMPLEX CARBOHYDRATES starches and fibre, which have a more complex chemical structure than sugars (known as simple carbohydrates).

ELIMINATION DIET a diet that excludes all but a very few foods in order to isolate food allergies or intolerances. Such a diet should be carried out only under medical supervision.

ENDORPHINS natural tranquillizers and painkillers that are produced in the brain in response to stress and strenuous exercise.

ENZYMES specific **proteins** that act as catalysts in chemical reactions that take place in the body. One of their functions is to aid digestion.

ESSENTIAL FATTY ACIDS [OMEGA-3 & OMEGA-6] unsaturated fats that are converted into prostaglandins which regulate white blood cells, thereby ensuring the proper functioning of the immune system. EFAs must be obtained through diet.

EXPECTORANT a substance that aids the expulsion of **mucus** and impurities from the lungs.

FIBRE a substance found in some fruits, vegetables and wholegrains, which aids digestion and can help prevent certain diseases.

FLAVONOIDS **phytonutrients** with **antioxidant** and antibacterial properties. They may protect against heart disease and some cancers.

FREE RADICALS atoms that are by-products of metabolism and can cause damage to cell membranes, leading to degenerative diseases, such as cancer. They can be neutralized by **antioxidants**.

FRUCTOSE natural fruit sugar.

GIARDIA an infection of the gut causing diarrhoea.

GLUTEN a protein found in wheat and other grains, such as barley, oats and rye.

HISTAMINE a substance released by the body in an allergic reaction that causes irritation.

INTERFERON a **protein** released by cells in order to inhibit the spread of viral infection.

LYMPHOCYTES white blood cells that carry out many different functions in the immune system.

MINERAL one of a group of essential nutrients required in small amounts for normal growth and development.

MUCOUS MEMBRANES the moist inner lining of the stomach, intestines, mouth, nasal sinuses and other parts of the body. They secrete mucus.

MUCUS a protective barrier or lubricant and a medium for carrying **enzymes**.

NATUROPATH a practitioner who treats disease without drugs, usually through diet, exercise, massage and other related techniques.

ORGANIC food produced without the routine use of pesticides, chemical fertilizers, herbicides, **antibiotics** or other growth promoters.

PATHOGEN an organism that causes disease.

PHAGOCYTE a cell capable of engulfing and absorbing foreign matter, thereby protecting the body from it.

PHYTONUTRIENTS bio-active compounds found in foods of plant origin that have health-enhancing qualities and protect us from disease. See chart on pages 139–40.

PROTEIN a macronutrient needed for growth, maintenance and repair by every cell in the body. The protein we eat is broken down into **amino acids**, which are then transported around the body via the bloodstream, and remade into specific proteins used by the body for a range of biological processes, such as cell repair and fighting infection.

REFINED FOODS refining foods results in loss of nutrients. Refined foods include white flour, white rice and white sugar.

SATURATED FAT a type of fatty acid that is usually solid at room temperature. It is the main type of fat in meat and dairy produce as well as in palm oil and coconut oil. Eating excessive amounts of saturated fat has been linked to an increased risk of heart disease.

TOFU soya bean curd that can be either "firm" or "silken". Firm tofu is the better form to use in stir-fries but silken tofu can be used for shakes and smoothies. Tofu is high in **protein** but low in fat, making it a healthy alternative to dairy products.

UNSATURATED FAT fats that are liquid at room temperature and form an important part of our diet. They can be divided into two groups: monounsaturated fat (found in olive oil, rapeseed oil, avocado and some nuts and seeds) and polyunsaturated fat (found in most vegetable oils, oily fish, and nuts and seeds and their oils).

VEGAN a diet that excludes meat, fish and any food derived from a living animal, including eggs and dairy produce.

VEGETARIAN Lacto-ovo vegetarians exclude red meat, poultry and fish from their diet; lacto vegetarians also exclude eggs.

VIRUS infectious micro-organisms that reproduce by invading another living cell. Viruses cause many diseases including the flu, the common cold, herpes and chicken pox.

VITAMIN one of a group of essential nutrients required in small amounts for normal growth and development. They cannot be manufactured by the body and must be acquired through diet.

WHOLEGRAIN The unrefined fruit or seed of a cereal. Wholegrain food has not had any of its nutrients removed.

ESSENTIAL NUTRIENTS

This chart lists the main nutrients needed by your child's body for optimum health, and gives details of the specific benefits offered by each nutrient and some of the foods in which they are found.

vitamin	benefits	good food sources
VITAMIN A	Anticarcinogenic; antioxidant; helps in the process of EFA metabolism; keeps vision healthy; protects skin	Butter, egg, liver, oily fish, vegetable margarine, whole milk
BETA-CAROTENE (plant-food source of vitamin A)	Antioxidant; protects skin and the lining of the intestines, lungs, nose and throat	All brightly-coloured fruits and vegetables, such as apricot, broccoli, cantaloupe melon, green leafy vegetables, mango, orange, red pepper, sweet potato
VITAMIN B1 (THIAMIN)	Aids metabolism; needed for growth and development	Brown rice, chickpea, liver, salmon, sunflower seed, wheatgerm, wholewheat flour
VITAMIN B2 (RIBOFLAVIN)	Needed for healthy skin and mucous membranes, and healthy growth and development	Almond, cucumber, egg, game, grape, liver, pea, poultry, yoghurt
VITAMIN B3 (NIACIN)	Anti-inflammatory; needed for the health of the digestive system and skin	Fish, liver, peanut, potato, poultry, soya bean, sunflower seed
VITAMIN B5 (PANTOTHENIC ACID)	Needed for the body's response to stress and the manufacture of antibodies	Avocado, corn, egg, lean meats, lentil, liver, mushroom, shellfish, wholegrain products
VITAMIN B6 (PYRIDOXINE)	Anti-inflammatory; needed for the body to build all cells, hormones and antibodies	Avocado, hazelnut, leek, lentil, rice, salmon, sunflower seed, tuna
VITAMIN B12	Needed for red blood cell formation; supports growth	Dairy products, egg, fish, lean meats, poultry, shellfish
FOLIC ACID	Needed for red blood cell production and the growth of healthy nerves, particularly in a developing foetus	Barley, blackberry, green leafy vegetables, liver, orange, pulses, spinach, wheatgerm
BIOTIN	Aids fat metabolism; helps the body to process carbohydrates, proteins, sugars and other vitamins	Brown rice, cashew nut, dairy products, egg, lentil, mackerel, mushroom, oats, poultry, sunflower seed, tuna
VITAMIN C	Anti-allergenic; antibacterial; anticarcinogenic; antihistamine; antioxidant; antiviral; improves wound healing; needed for EFA metabolism	Blackcurrant, broccoli, citrus fruits, green pepper, guava, kale, kiwi fruit, parsley, watercress
VITAMIN D	Helps control the use of calcium; needed for strong bones and teeth	Egg, herring, mackerel, salmon, sardine, shiitake mushroom
VITAMIN E	Antioxidant; helps to protect skin, circulation, brain and hormones against pollution; needed for efficient antibody response to infection	Almond, avocado, butternut squash, oatmeal, sunflower oil and seed, sweet potato, walnut
VITAMIN K	Needed to ensure normal blood clotting	Cabbage, cauliflower, cheese, green tea, oats, pea, soya bean
mineral		
CALCIUM	Builds healthy bones; helps EFA metabolism	Almond, calcium-enriched soya products (such as tofu), green leafy vegetables, kale, molasses, sardine, soya milk and yoghurt, tahini, yoghurt
COPPER	Needed in tiny amounts to transport red blood cells around the body	Barley, cashew nut, lentil, molasses, mussels, oats, salmon, walnut

mineral	benefits	good food sources
IRON	Needed to carry oxygen around the body, and for the production of white blood cells and antibodies	Chickpea, dried apricot, egg yolk, game, green leafy vegetables, lentil, liver, molasses, red meat, sardine, wholegrains
MAGNESIUM	Needed for antibody production, EFA metabolism and the growth and development of bones	Dried fruits, fish, green leafy vegetables, nuts and seeds, wholegrain cereals
MANGANESE	Antioxidant	Avocado, barley, blackberry, buckwheat, ginger, oats, pea, pulses, seaweed
POTASSIUM	Boosts energy and strength; helps to prevent water retention	Avocado, banana, blackberry, citrus fruits, lentil, molasses, nuts, parsnip, raisin, spinach, wholegrains
SELENIUM	Anticarcinogenic; antioxidant; helps to produce antibodies	Brazil nut, celery, courgette, garlic, mushroom, onion, pumpkin seed, seafood, sesame seed, sunflower seed
SULPHUR	Aids bile secretion in liver; antioxidant	Cabbage, egg, fish, garlic, onion, wheatgerm
ZINC	Antioxidant; needed for EFA metabolism, wound healing and for growth and regeneration of white blood cells	Game, molasses, poultry, shellfish, sunflower seed, wholegrains

other important nutrients	benefits	good food sources
ESSENTIAL FATTY ACIDS (EFAS)	Needed for brain power, healthy nerves, smooth skin, hormone balance and to help prevent inflammation	Linseed oil, nuts, oily fish (such as herring, mackerel, salmon, sardine), pumpkin, sesame oil and seed, sunflower oil and seed

GUIDE TO PHYTONUTRIENTS

Phytonutrients are biologically-active compounds that are found in plant foods. In recent years, research into phytonutrients and their possible health benefits has become an important part of nutrition research. It is still an emerging science, however, and there is a long way to go before we properly understand their role in the prevention of disease. To date, around 12,000 phytonutrients have been identified, of which several have been recognized as being particularly beneficial to human health. Throughout this book you will have encountered many phytonutrients. The chart below lists those most commonly cited, their possible health benefits and the top foods in which they can be found. Please note that beta-carotene is categorized as a vitamin in the food listings' immune profiles as it can be converted by the body into the essential vitamin A.

carotenoids	possible benefits	good food sources
ALPHA-CAROTENE		Avocado, carrot, red pepper, squash, sweetcorn, tomato
BETA-CAROTENE	All carotenoids are anticarcinogenic; antioxidant; maintain healthy skin; protect vision; support a healthy heart	All brightly-coloured fruits and vegetables, such as apricot, broccoli, cantaloupe melon, kale, mango, orange, parsley, red pepper, spinach, sweet potato, watercress
CRYPTOXANTHIN		Guava, mango, nectarine, orange, papaya, passionfruit, peach, red pepper, tangerine
LUTEIN		Blackcurrant, broccoli, butternut squash, kale, kiwi fruit, lettuce, pea, spinach, spring greens, sweetcorn
LYCOPENE		Apricot, guava, pink grapefruit, tomato
ZEAXANTHIN		Butternut squash, cos lettuce, orange, spinach, spring greens, sweetcorn

flavonoids	possible benefits	good food sources
ANTHOCYANINS		Aubergine, blackberry, blackcurrant, black grape, blueberry, cherry, cranberry, elderberry, pear, raspberry, strawberry
CATECHINS	All flavonoids are antibacterial; anticarcinogenic; anti-inflammatory; antioxidant; antiviral; blood cleansing	Apple, cocoa, grape, pear
HESPERIDIN		Citrus fruits and rind
PROANTHOCYANIDINS		Apple, blackcurrant, black-eyed bean, cherry, cranberry, grape, kidney bean, lentil, pear
QUERCETIN		Apple, broad bean, grape, kale, lemon rind, lollo rosso lettuce, olive, onion, tomato
RUTIN		Buckwheat, cabbage, green bean, oats, pea
other useful phytonutrients		
ALLIUM COMPOUNDS (such as allicin)	Antibacterial; antifungal; antiparasitic; antiviral	Chive, garlic, leek, onion
CAPSAICIN	Analgesic; anti-inflammatory; antiseptic	Chilli, turmeric
CHLOROPHYLL	Anticarcinogenic	Any green vegetable
COUMARINS	Anticarcinogenic; antioxidant	Celery, citrus fruits, coriander, fennel, parsley, parsnip
COUMESTROL	Anticarcinogenic	Alfafa sprout, mung beansprout
CURCUMIN	Anticarcinogenic; anti-inflammatory	Sweetcorn, turmeric
ELLAGIC ACID	Anticarcinogenic	Blackberry, blueberry, cherry, cranberry, raspberry, strawberry, walnut
ISOFLAVONES	Anticarcinogenic; protects against heart disease	Lentil, millet, soya bean and soya products such as miso, soya milk, tempeh and tofu
ISOTHIOCYANATES	Anticarcinogenic	Broccoli, Brussels sprout, cabbage
LENTINAN	Anticarcinogenic; antiviral	Shiitake mushroom
LIGNANS	Anticarcinogenic	Barley, linseed, oats, pumpkin seed, rye, sesame seed, sunflower seed, wholewheat
LIMINOIDS	Anticarcinogenic	Citrus fruits and rind
LIMONENE	Anticarcinogenic	Citrus fruits and rind, mint
PHYTIC ACID	Anticarcinogenic; antioxidant	Lentil, seeds and nuts, wholegrains
PROTEASE INHIBITORS	Anticarcinogenic; protects against heart disease	Wholegrains such as barley, chickpea, lentil, oats, rye, soya bean, wheat
RESVERATOL	Anticarcinogenic; antioxidant; protects against heart disease	Grape skin, mulberry, peanut
SAPONINS	Antibacterial; anticarcinogenic; antiparasitic	Beans, chickpea, garlic, mung beansprout, oats, quinoa

index

NOTE: Page numbers for main descriptions are given in bold. The index should be used in conjunction with the glossary (see pages 136–7), the guide to phytonutrients (see pages 139–40) and the cross-references from the individual food listings in Part Two to the recipes elsewhere in the book.

a

adaptive immune system 11
additives 102, 110, 121
adenoids 12, 124
AIDS/HIV 20, 24–5, 55
ajoene 57
alfalfa sprouts **37**, 128
allergens 11, 114
allergies and allergic reactions 11, **15**, 29, 31, **114–15**, 120
  see also hay fever *and* migraine
  and asthma 102
  and coeliac disease 132
  and ear infections 127
  and eczema 112
  foods likely to cause 35, 41, 44, 45, 102, 114, 118, 127
allicin 56, 57
allium family **22** *see also* garlic, leek *and* onion
almond **36**, 102, 108, 112, 113, 114, 118, 120, 128, 129, 130, 132
amaranth **40**, 132
anaemia 21, 47
analgesics 53, 102
anchovy **44**, 121
animals 11, 102, 112
anti-inflammatories *see* inflammation
antibiotics **13–14**, 51, 104, 125, 126–7
antibodies 11
antihistamines 118–19
  see also histamine
antioxidants (*main references only*) 13, 84, 92
  amounts needed 91
  colour as guide to levels 103
antiseptics 53, 55
appendix 12
apple **30–31**, 114, 128, 130, 132, 134
apple cider vinegar 112, 113
apricot **27**, **33**, 106, 108, 110, 112, 114, 116, 124, 128, 132
arginine 111, 117
arthritis 15, 29, 32, 39, 44
asparagus 128
aspirin 102
asthma **102–3**, 114, 115
autoimmune diseases 15, 132

avenin 43, 133
avocado **18**, 110, 112, 116, 121

b

B-lymphocytes 11
B-vitamins 12, 23, 46–7, 84, 92, 103, 104, 113, **138**
babies 10, 60–61, 68
bacon 121
bacteria *see also* candida
  and antibiotics 13–14, 104
  beneficial 10, 50–51, 57, 104
  for yoghurt 50
bacterial infections 13–14, 124
baked bean 130
baking, recipes for 63, 66, 83, 90, 91, 99, 133
banana **31**, 110, 116, 121, 132, 134
barley **40**, 110, 116, 118, 124
baths 108, 113
beans **52**, 104, 111, 117, 128, 130, 132 *see also* soya
  sprouted **37**, 110, 116, 128
beetroot **18**, 108, 110, 116, 126
bell pepper *see* peppers
berries **27**, **30**, 108, 109, 110, 114, 116, 118, 121, 126, 130, 132
beta-carotene (*main references only*) 19, 20–21, 123, **138**
bile 12
bio-yoghurt 50
biotin 47, **138**
biscuits, recipes for 39, 43, 91
bites 11
blackberry **27**, 118
blackcurrant **28–9**, 102, 108, 109, 110, 114, 116, 118, 120, 124, 125, 135
blood cells 11, 12, 110, 111
blood clots 57
blood sugar levels 120, 130, 131
blueberry **27**, 108, 109, 110, 114, 116, 118, 126, 135
bok choi **22**, 114, 124
bone marrow 12
bottle-feeding 60, 61, 109, 113, 127, 132
brain function 39, 48
brazil nut 128, 132
bread 130, 134

recipes for 63, 95, 105
  yeast-free 105
breakfast 84–5, 93
  recipes for 62, 78, 86, 94
breastfeeding and breast milk 10, 11, 60, 61, 112, 113, 115, 127, 134
  mother's diet 60, 61, 62–6
broccoli **20–21**, 102, 103, 106, 110, 114, 116, 118, 120, 124, 128, 130, 132
bromelain 32
bronchitis 54, 57
brown lentil *see* lentil
brown rice *see* rice
buckwheat **40**, 114, 118, 132
burgers 86, 88
burnt food *see under* food(s)
butter bean **52**, 130
butternut squash *see under* squash

c

cabbage 20, **23**, 106, 114, 118, 130
caffeine 120, 121
cakes, recipes for 66, 83, 133
calcium 12, 26, 41, 51, 77, **138**
camomile 120, 121, 135
cancer 24, **128–9**
  protection against 18, 21, 22, 23, 24, 27, 30, 31, 32, 35, 36, 37, 40, 43, 45, 52, 53, 54, 55, 56, 129
  substances causing risk of 35, 68
candida (*Candida Albicans*) 57, **104–5**
cantaloupe melon **31**, 108, 112, 114, 126, 132
capsaicin 53
capsicums *see* peppers
carbohydrates 84–5
carotenoids 21, 29
carrot **19**, 102, 104, 106, 108, 110, 112, 114, 116, 120, 124, 126, 128, 132, 134, 135
cashew nut **36**, 108, 120, 130, 132
catarrh 53 *see also* mucus
cauliflower **23**, 128, 130
celery 106, 126

cereals **40–43** *see also* individual cereals
cheese 111, 117, 121
chemicals 12
cherry **27**, 120
chicken **44**, 106, 107, 109, 124, 126, 135
chicken pox 108–9
chickpea **52**, 130
chicory 128
chilli **53**, 102, 106, 119, 120, 126, 135
chive **22**
chlorophyll 32, 53
chocolate 111, 117, 121
cholesterol 35, 48, 52, 57
chronic fatigue syndrome **110–11**
cigarette smoke 13, 102, 127
cinnamon **53**, 102, 106, 107, 108, 119
citrus fruits 106, 108, 113
  see also individual fruits
clementine 35
clove **53**, 102, 107
cod **44**
coeliac disease 43, **132–3**
colds 14, 19, 21, 53, 57, 76, 106, 124, **135**
  and asthma 102
colitis 15, 44
collagen 20
complex carbohydrates 84–5
concentration 93
condiments **53–7**
constipation 19, 31, 40, 52
copper **138**
coriander 53
corn (sweetcorn) **26**, **40**, 132
coughs 53, **106–7**
courgette 106
cranberry **27**
Crohn's disease 15
curcumin 26, 55
currant 28

d

dairy products **50–51**, 77, 106, 111, 112, 118, 121, 125, 127, 129, 134 *see also* cheese, egg *and* yoghurt
date **33**

dehydration 120, 123, 124, 134, 135
dermatitis *see* eczema
design a bug 82
detergents 112
diabetes 15, 21, 76, **130–31**
diarrhoea 19, 31, 60, **134**
digestion and digestive system
    10, 11, 32, 130
    tonics for 53
digestive problems 27, 40
    see also coeliac disease
dips 21, 57, 96
dried fruits **33**, 132
dried pulses **52**
drinks 76, 93, 103, 109, 119,
    124, 135 *see also* smoothies
    rehydration 134, 135
duck **47**, 110, 116
dust 11, 102, 124
dust mites 102, 112
dyslexia 48
dyspraxia 48

e
ear infections 57, **126–7**
echinacea 109, 135
E. coli 29
eczema 44, 102, **112–13**, 114,
    115
EFAs *see* essential fatty acids
egg **45**, 106, 108, 110, 111,
    113, 114, 117, 130
elimination diets 112, 115
ellagic acid 27, 30
encephalitis 120
energy 84, 85, 93
Epstein-Barr virus 110, 111, 116,
    117
essential fatty acids (EFAs) 36,
    38–9, 42, 44, 45, 48, 113,
    115, **139**
essential oils 106
eucalyptus 106
Eustachian tube 126, 127
evening primrose oil 61, 112,
    113, 115, 128
exclusion diets 112, 115, 120, 121
exercise 12, 102, 131
eyes 120

f
farming practices 14, 35, 47, 48
fasting **134**
fat levels 48, 61, 131
fatigue 84, 110
fennel 106, 120
fever 116, 123, 124, **135**
fig 118
fingernails 47

fish **44–5**, **48–9**, 111, 113, 114,
    117, 121 *see also*
    individual fish
fish farming 48, 49
fizzy drinks 76, 93
flavonoids 28–9, 35
flaxseed *see* linseed
flu 14, 53, 57, 110
fluids *see* drinks
folic acid 47, **138**
food(s)
    allergies to *see* allergies
    antibiotics in 14
    burnt 13, 84
    fried 13, 84, 106
    non-organic 14, 35, 47, 48, 68
    organic 68
    processed 110
    raw 68
    refined 107, 131
    variety necessary 115
food additives 102, 110, 121
food intolerance 114–15
    see also allergies
food poisoning 55
formula milks 60, 61, 109, 113, 134
free radicals (*main references
    only*) 13, 84
fried food *see under* food(s)
fructose **54**, 130
fruit **27–35**, 85 *see also*
    individual fruits
    colour as guide to antioxidant
    content 103
fruit smoothies *see* smoothies
fruit yoghurt 50, 51
fungicides 35

g
game **46–7**, 112, 114, 120, 132
garlic **22**, **56–7**, 102, 104, 106,
    107, 108, 109, 110, 111, 114,
    116, 117, 118, 119, 120, 124,
    125, 126, 128, 130, 135
    ear drops 126
gastroenteritis 40
giardia 57, 60
ginger **54**, 102, 103, 106, 107,
    108, 118, 119, 120, 121, 126,
    128, 135
glandular fever 40, 110, **116–17**
glucose 54, 130
gluten 40, 43, 112, 132, 133
golden seal 109, 135
gooseberry 28
grains *see* cereals
grape **30**, 124
grapefruit **32**, 118, 126, 135
green bean 104

green cabbage *see* cabbage
green leafy vegetables 104, 112
    see also individual vegetables
green lentil *see* lentil
green tea 106, 128
groats 43
guava 28, **31**, 108, 126, 135
gum infections 53
gut, bacteria in 10, 104–5

h
hair–mineral analysis 113
ham 121
hay fever **118–19**
headaches 55, **120–21**, 135
heart 21, 30, 48, 57, 131
hedgehog, mango 83
herbs **53–5**, 109
herpes group of viruses 40, 108,
    110, 111
herring 48, 102, 104, 112
hesperidin 35
histamine 11, 29, 114, 121
    see also antihistamines
HIV/AIDS 20, 24–5, 55
honey **54**, 106, 107, 118, 120
    locally produced 119
hormones 92
horseradish 102, 106, 118, 119,
    126, 135
hospitals 14
hummus 21
hyperactivity 48, 115
hyperglycaemia 130
hypoglycaemia 120

i
ice cream 83
ice pops 107, 109, 116, 123, 125
IgA/IgD/IgE/IgG/IgM 11, 60
immune system 10–12
    development 10, 14, 60, 68,
    76, 84
    and fever 135
    and nutrients 12–13
immunization (vaccination) 15, 122
immunity 10
immunoglobulins *see* antibodies
infections *see* viruses and viral
    infections
inflammation and anti-
    inflammatories 26, 29, 32, 39,
    44, 55, 115
innate immune system 11
insect bites and stings 11
insulin 130, 131
interferon 24, 28, 111, 117
intestine 12, 57, 132
iron 12, 21, 26, 33, 47, 92, **139**

and vitamin C 34
irritants 112

k
kale **26**, 110, 114, 116, 118,
    120, 124, 128, 130
ketchup 121
kidney bean 130
kissing babies 61
kiwi fruit **32**, 108, 110, 116, 126

l
lactic acid 50
lactose 50, 134
lassi 51
lavender 106, 120
learning difficulties 48
leek **22**, 104, 106
lemon 28, **31**, 102, 106, 118,
    124, 126, 135
lentil **52**, 128, 130, 132
lentinan 24, 25, 111, 117
lettuce **18**, 106, 110, 116, 124,
    128, 130, 132
lime 102, 106, 118, 124, 126, 135
liminoids 31
limonene 31, 35, 54
linoleic acid 42
linseed, and linseed oil
    36, 61, 112, 113, 120, 128, 132
live yoghurt 50, 104, 105, 125
liver 12, 116–17
lutein 29
lycopene 32
lymphatic system 11–12
lymphocytes 11–12
lysine 40, 111, 117

m
mackerel **45**, 102, 104, 112, 118
macrophages 11
magnesium 12, 92, 102–3, 111,
    113, **139**
main meals, recipes for 62–6,
    79–82, 86–90, 94–8
maize (sweetcorn) **26**, **40**, 132
mandarin 34
manganese **139**
mango **32**, 102, 106, 108, 110,
    112, 116, 124, 126, 128, 132
manuka honey **54**, 106, 107
meals and mealtimes 76, 85, 93
measles **122–3**
meat **44**, **46–7**, 106, 121, 129
melon **31**, 108, 112, 114, 126, 132
meningitis 120, 135
menstruation 92
menu planners 61, 69, 77, 85, 93
migraine 115, **120–21**

milk 76, 113, 114, 115
    see also dairy products
milks, formula 60, 61, 109, 113, 134
millet **40**, 102, 104, 114, 120, 124, 132
mint **54**
molasses **54**, 132
mononucleosis *see* glandular fever
moulds 11, 102
mucous membranes 10
mucus 44, 53, 54, 57, 106, 125, 127
muesli 72, 86, 94
mushroom 25 *see also* shiitake mushroom
myalgic encephalomyelitis, or ME (chronic fatigue syndrome) **110–11**

n

natural killer (NK) cells 11
nectarine **30**
niacin *see* vitamin B3
NK (natural killer) cells 11
nursing mothers 60
nutritionists and nutritional therapists 112, 113
nuts 36, **38–9**, 109, 111, 112, 114, 117, 121, 128, 132
    see also individual nuts
    storing 39

o

oat bran 130
oatcakes 43
oats **42–3**, 108, 112, 130, 133
obesity 76, 131
oestrogen 92
oils 48, 112, 113 *see also* essential oils
    evening primrose oil 61, 112, 113, 115, 128
    linseed oil **36**, 61, 112, 113
    olive oil 104, 120, 128
    walnut oil 39
oily fish **44–5**, **48–9**, 113
    see also individual fish
olive oil 104, 120, 128
omega-3 EFAs 38–9, 44, 45, 48
omega-6 EFAs 38–9, 42
onion **22**, 104, 106, 108, 114, 118, 120, 124, 126, 135
orange 20, **34–5**, 106, 110, 116, 118, 121, 124, 126, 130, 135
oregano 135
organic food *see under* food(s)

p

painkillers 53, 102
pantothenic acid *see* vitamin B5
papaya **32**, 102, 106, 108, 110, 116, 124, 135
parasites and parasitic infections 57, 60
parsley **54–5**, 102, 106, 108, 110, 116, 120, 126, 135
parsley, Chinese *see* coriander
parsnip **22**
passive immunity 10, 60
pasta 130, 131
paw paw *see* papaya
peach 30
peanut 130
pear **31**, 114, 120, 130, 132
pearl barley 40
pea **26**, 128, 132, 135
pectin 30–31, 35
peppermint **54**
peppers **19**, 102, 114, 124
    see also chilli
pesticides 12, 48, 68
pesto 39
pets 11, 102, 112
phytic acid 37, 40, 43
phytonutrients (*main references only*) 13, 139–40
phytosterols 37
pine nut **36**
pineapple **32**, 120, 135
pink grapefruit **32**
pizza 80
    potato-based 105
placenta 10, 11
plum 121
pollen 11, 102, 118
    and locally produced honey 119
pollution 12, 13, 44, 48, 49, 84, 102
popcorn **40**
porridge 78
porridge oats 43
posture 120
pot barley **40**
potassium **139**
potato **22**, 121, 132
poultry 111, 117, 132
prawn **45**
pregnancy 10, 11, 60
probiotics 51, 61, 105, 125
prostaglandins 48
protein 41, 42, 52, 84–5
puberty 92
puddings, recipes for 66, 75, 82–3, 90–91, 98–9
pulses **52**, 128
pumpkin 106, 112, 114, 126

pumpkin seed **36–7**, 108, 110, 112, 113, 114, 116, 128, 130, 132
purées 68, 69, 70–73
purple sprouting broccoli 21
pyridoxine *see* vitamin B6

q

quercetin 31
quinoa **41**, 102, 104, 114, 124, 128, 132

r

radiation 13
raisin **33**, 132
raspberry 108, 121, 132
raw foods *see under* food(s)
red cabbage *see* cabbage
red lentil *see* lentil
red pepper *see* peppers
refined foods *see under* food(s)
rehydration drinks 134
respiratory complaints 44, 57
    see also asthma
respiratory system 10–11
retinol 19, 109, 123
rheumatoid arthritis 15, 44
rhinitis *see* hay fever
riboflavin *see* vitamin B2
rice **40**, 102, 104, 106, 110, 114, 116, 118, 120, 124, 128, 130, 132
rice cakes 134
rice milk 134
rocket 118, 120
rolled oats 43
rosemary **55**, 118
rye 130

s

safflower oil 48, 113
sage 135
salads and dressings 81, 98, 117
salami 121
saliva 11
salmon **48–9**, 102, 103, 104, 110, 112, 113, 114, 116, 118, 128
salt 106
saponins 52
sardine 104, 118, 121
sauerkraut 121
sausage 121
school 84, 92, 93
school food 84
seafood 130, 132 *see also* fish *and* shellfish
seeds **36–7**, 109, 112, 121
    sprouted **37**

selenium 12, 36, 45, **139**
semen 92
sesame seed **37**, 114, 128, 130, 132
shallot **22**
shellfish 114
shiitake mushroom **24–5**, 110, 111, 116, 117, 126, 128
silicon 40
sinus problems 53, 54, 119
skin 10
smoking 13, 102, 127
smoothies 35, 36, 43, 66, 83, 91, 94, 99, 109, 117, 131
snacks 76, 85, 93
soap 112
soda bread 95, 105
solids, introducing *see* weaning
sore throat 31, 116, **124–5**
soups 25, 35, 40, 47, 62–3, 80, 95, 103, 111, 123, 127, 135
soya bean 48, **52**, 114, 130
    see also tofu
    sprouted **37**
soya milk 128
soya yoghurt 50, 51, 105
spices **53–5**, 103 *see also individual spices*
spinach **26**, 121
spirulina 130
spleen 12
sprouted seeds/beans **37**, 110, 116, 128
sprout (Brussels sprout) 128
squash **26**, 102, 108, 110, 112, 114, 116, 124, 135
squid **45**
stings 11
stomach 10, 57
stomach upsets 27, 29, 40
strawberry **30**, 108, 132
Streptococcus 124
stress 76, 84, 92, 102, 112, 120
sugar 104, 105, 106, 107, 121
    fructose **54**, 130
sulphur **139**
sulphur dioxide 33
sunflower seed, and sunflower oil **37**, 48, 102, 108, 110, 112, 113, 114, 116, 128, 130, 132
supper 85
sweat 10
sweat tests 113
sweet pepper *see* peppers
sweet potato **22**, 106, 108, 110, 112, 114, 116, 124, 126, 128, 132, 135
sweetcorn **26**, **40**, 132

t

T-helpers 11
T-lymphocytes 11
T-suppressors 11
tahini **37**
tangerine 34, 35
tea, green 106, 128
tea tree (manuka) honey **54**, 106, 107
tears 10, 11
teenagers 92–3
thiamine *see* vitamin B1
throat infections 19 *see also* sore throat
thyme **55**, 102, 106, 107, 118, 135
thymus 12
tiredness 84, 110
tobacco 13, 102, 126
tofu 108, 111, 117, 126, 128
tomato **18**, 110, 113, 116, 121, 128, 132
tomato ketchup 121
tonsillitis 124
tonsils 12, 124
tooth infections 53
tuna **44**, 102, 104, 110, 112, 116, 121
turkey **44**, 124
turmeric **55**, 118, 119, 128
turnip 118
tyramine 121

u

ulcerative colitis 15, 44
urinary infections/problems 27, 29, 40, 53
urine 10, 12

v

vaccination 15, 122
vegan/dairy-free diets 7, 26
vegetables **18–26** *see also individual vegetables*
    colour as guide to antioxidant content 103
venison **47**, 110, 116
vinegar 112, 113
viruses and viral infections 13–14, 21, 76, 124, 135 *see also* colds *and* glandular fever
    and asthma 102
    and chronic fatigue syndrome 110
    and development of immune system 10, 76
    and eczema 112
    herpes group 40, 108, 110, 111
    mutations 135
vitamin A 12, 19, 45, 109, 122–3, **138**
vitamin B *see* B-vitamins *and following entries*
vitamin B1 (thiamine) 46, **138**
vitamin B2 (riboflavin) 46, **138**
vitamin B3 (niacin) 23, 46, **138**
vitamin B5 (pantothenic acid) 46, **138**
vitamin B6 (pyridoxine) 46–7, 92, **138**
vitamin B12 47, **138**
vitamin C (*main references only*) 12, 20, 23, 27, 28, 103, 113, 135, **138**
    and iron 34
vitamin D 25, **138**
vitamin E 12, **138**
vitamin K **138**
vomiting **134**

w

walnut **38–9**, 108, 113
watercress **19**, 102, 106, 118, 120, 124
watermelon **30**, 132, 135
waxing of fruit 35
weaning 31, 68–9, 112–13, 114, 115
wheat **41**, 104, 113, 114, 115, 118, 121, 130
    alternatives to 26, 40, 41, 118
wheatgerm **41**
white blood cells 11, 12, 110, 111
whooping cough 57

y

yeast 104–5
yeast extract 121
yoghurt **50–51**, 104, 105, 125, 130
    homemade 51, 82

z

zinc 12, 36–7, 92, 113, 123, 135, **139**
    deficiency symptoms 47
zucchini *see* courgette

bibliography

Academic Press, *Encyclopedia of Foods* (Academic Press, US, 2001)

Balch, Phyllis and James F. Balch, *Prescription for Nutritional Healing* (Avery Publishing, US, 2002)

Brostoff, Dr Jonathan, and Linda Gamlin, *The Complete Guide to Allergy and Intolerance* (Bloomsbury Press, UK, 1998)

Burney, Lucy, *Optimum Nutrition for Babies and Young Children* (Piatkus Books, UK, 1999)

Burney, Lucy, *Boost Your Child's Immune System* (Piatkus Books, UK, 2001)

Clark, Susan, *What Really Works for Kids* (Bantam Press, US, 2003)

Cousin, Jean Pierre, *Food is Medicine* (Duncan Baird Publishers, UK, 2002)

Davidson, Alan, *The Oxford Companion to Food* (Oxford University Press, UK, 1999)

Davies, Dr Stephen, and Dr Alan Stewart, *Nutritional Medicine* (Pan Books, UK, 1987)

Elliott, Rose and Carlo de Paoli, *The Kitchen Pharmacy* (Orion publishing, UK, 1998)

Erasmus, Udo, *Fats that Heal and Fats that Kill* (Alive Books, Canada, 1998)

Ewin, Jeanette, *The Plants We Need to Eat* (Thorsons, UK, 1997)

Hartvig, Kirsten, *Eat for Immunity* (Duncan Baird Publishers, UK, 2003

Holford, Patrick, *The Optimum Nutrition Bible* (Piatkus Books, UK, 1998)

Kiple, Kenneth F, and Conee Ornelas Krienhild (Eds.), *The Cambridge World History of Food* (Cambridge University Press, UK, 2000)

Lininger, Schuyler W., *The Natural Pharmacy* (Prima Publishing, US, 1999)

MacCance and Widdowson, *The Composition of Foods Sixth Summary Edition* (the Royal Society of Chemistry and the Food Standards Agency, UK, 2002)

MacGregor, Janet, *An Introduction to the Anatomy and Physiology of Children* (Routledge, Taylor and Francis Group, UK and US, 1999)

Murray, Michael, and Joseph Pizzorno, *Encyclopedia of Natural Medicine* (Random House, UK and US, 2001)

Reader's Digest, *Foods that Harm, Foods that Heal* (Reader's Digest, UK, 2002)

Sompayrac, Lauren M., *How the Immune System Works* (Blackwell Science, US, 2003)

Thompson, Joyce M., *Nutritional Requirements of Infants and Young Children* (Blackwell Science, UK, 1997)

Van Stratten, Michael and Barbara Griggs, *Superfoods* (Dorling Kindersley, UK, 1990)

Werbach, Melvyn R, M.D., *Nutritional Influences on Illness* (Third Line Press, US, 1996)